AIDS

ALSO BY ELISABETH KÜBLER-ROSS

On Death and Dying

Questions and Answers on Death and Dying

To Live Until We Say Good-Bye

Living With Death and Dying

Remember the Secret

Death: The Final Stage of Growth

On Children and Death

Working It Through

ELISABETH KÜBLER-ROSS, M.D.

AIDS
The Ultimate Challenge

Macmillan Publishing Company   *New York*
Collier Macmillan Publishers   *London*

Macmillan Publishing Company
866 Third Avenue, New York, N.Y. 10022
Collier Macmillan Canada, Inc.

Library of Congress Cataloging-in-Publication Data
Kübler-Ross, Elisabeth, M.D.
  AIDS: the ultimate challenge.
  Includes index.
  1. AIDS (Disease)—Palliative treatment. 2. AIDS
(Disease)—Psychological aspects. 3. Terminal care.
I. Title.   [DNLM: 1. Acquired Immunodeficiency
Syndrome—popular works. 2. Terminal Care—popular
works. WD 308 K95a]
RC607.A26K83 1987   616.97'92   87-24016
ISBN 0-02-567170-7

Macmillan books are available at special discounts for bulk purchases for sales promotions, premiums, fund-raising, or educational use. For details, contact:

Special Sales Director
Macmillan Publishing Company
866 Third Avenue
New York, N.Y. 10022

10 9 8 7 6 5 4 3 2 1

Printed in the United States of America

This book is dedicated to G., who lived only nine months but whose life was not in vain. And to Larry. And to all our AIDS patients—the men, women, and children—who, through their suffering, became our teachers in *love,* understanding, and compassion.

—*Elisabeth*

"Today, something is happening to the whole structure of human consciousness. A fresh kind of life is starting."

—*Teilhard de Chardin*

Contents

Acknowledgments

Credit has to be given to the best secretary I have ever had in the twenty years of needing office help and assistance in typing my fourteen books. Frances Luthy has not only run my office in my many absences and seen to it that my mail was always taken care of, but she has—in an untiring way—transcribed my whole manuscript during long nights and weekends and given every help to meet the deadline for the printing of this book.

Robert Stewart, my editor, has done more for me and the birth of this book than any other editor I ever had. He spent several days at my farm and worked through many a night to put the final touches on this manuscript. Thanks to both of these marvelous helpers and friends.

To my two triplet sisters, who have contributed in their unique ways: Erika, through sending me an endless supply of Swiss chocolates to keep me going during the months this book was written, and Eva, for joining me temporarily at the farm and supervising my volunteer staff and by constantly reminding me to celebrate life every day in the midst of this "death and dying" work.

Also, my deep *danke dir* goes to Evelyn, who came from Germany to keep up my harvesting and canning, as well as my two Swiss farmers who tended to my animals and land while I "hid in the mountains" to complete this work.

There were naturally people whose contributions made this book possible, the AIDS patients themselves, the many mothers and children who shared their stories, the inmates from different institutions, Nancy and Bob Alexander, who visit them weekly, and my special friend, Irene Smith, whose work has enriched many lives on the West Coast and whose growth has been an example to many a despairing soul. She is an example for any faint-hearted person and her example will be the shining light to thousands, who, in the future, will venture out into the field of loving service to those stricken with AIDS.

Thank you Mwalimu Imara, you have stuck it out with me for twenty years, starting as one of my theology students two decades ago and going over my first book, *On Death and Dying,* and again you are the first person to read the complete manuscript of this, my fourteenth book.

Thank you, thank you, thank you, and bless you all.

—Elisabeth

AIDS

Introduction

It may be necessary to give those readers who are unfamiliar with what I do a brief summary of my life's work so they will understand why working with AIDS patients was a natural outgrowth of my everyday work and concern.

For over twenty years I have been involved in caring for terminally ill patients, both adults and children. My goal has been, and still is, to educate health-care professionals as well as clergy to become more familiar with the needs, concerns, fears, and anxieties of individuals (and their families) who face the end of their lives.

As a result of my work with medical and theological students at the University of Chicago, and hundreds of terminally ill patients who volunteered to be interviewed by me for their "enlightenment," my first book, *On Death and Dying,* was published in 1969. It was in that book that I explain the "stages of dying"—*denial and isolation, anger, bargaining, depression,* and *acceptance*—simply outlining the major emotional reactions patients, family, and sometimes even hospital staff undergo from the beginning of the diagnosis of a potentially fatal illness up to the death of the patient. Those five stages have been found again and again (not necessarily in the same chronological order) in many different forms of loss besides critical illness: in couples who go through divorce or separation; in a family whose house burns down; a farmer who loses his farm to bankruptcy; in parents whose child ends up in jail instead of college; mothers whose sons are found to be drug addicts or pushers.

Depending on the personality of the individual and/ or the suddenness of the occurring drama, the stages of dying, as we used to call them two decades ago, can surface dramatically and quickly. In the sudden death of a child, however, many a parent stays in a state of shock, numbness, and denial for weeks. It can even last for years if in the emergency room or trauma unit the parents are sedated and tranquilized when the news is given, if they are stuffed with Valium to block emotional reactions and are sent home without the chance to view the body. As I've said elsewhere, health-care givers have to become more honest; we have to admit that we use far too many tranquilizers, that we send families home only half aware of the reality of their loss. The result is a prolonged and painful mourning period that is easily preventable.

We have, in many of our workshops, strongly advocated that soundproof "screaming rooms" be established adjacent to emergency rooms, and that they be staffed by members of the Compassionate Friends, who have worked through their own grief over the death of a child and can thereby help newly bereaved families exter-

2

nalize their pain, disbelief, anger, and rage before returning home. In this way they will have already begun to deal with their loss and be better able to inform the rest of the family and friends, share the death of a child with a sibling, and prepare for the funeral.

Life was tough in the early days. There was so much resistance, so much fear and reluctance. Many thought it "odd," or at least unworthy of a physician, that one would spend so much time with dying patients. It was very difficult to obtain permission from primary physicians for medical and theology students to interview their dying patients. The doctors were afraid they might become "famous" for their dying patients—their "failures"—rather than for their successes. Cancer was a word that few mentioned openly in those days, and substitute labels such as "tumor" and "growth" were used when a patient inquired about the results of tests and examinations.

More often than not the family was informed but not the patient whose life was threatened by the diagnosis of a malignancy. Two decades later, laws and attitudes have changed. Thousands of books and papers written on the topic of terminal illness have led to yet another subspecialty, thanatology. Patients and families now talk more about an impending death, and thousands are preparing their own funerals. By accepting their deaths, patients are more willing to finalize their Last Will and Testament to ensure that their wishes are known and the family taken care of. There is rarely a medical or nursing school, a seminary, or social work institution where courses are not given on the needs of terminally ill patients. The clergy have also come a long way in their counseling.

Hospices have sprung up in every major area and palliative care units are available. Dying patients and their families now have several alternatives to dying in a regular hospital. Thanks largely to the thousands of classes, workshops, and seminars given at medical and nursing schools, theological seminaries, and social work schools all over the country—many using *On Death and Dying* as their textbook—families are given the option of taking dying family members home for the final stage of their illness. When the science of medicine has done all it can, patients can either sign themselves into a palliative care unit or a hospice, where the quality of life is emphasized and not the prolongation of dying (at all costs!).

Hundreds of hospices are now available throughout the United States and overseas, and a couple of years ago we proudly started the Children's Hospice International, Inc., an umbrella organization to facilitate the inclusion of children in regular hospices as well as to establish hospices for children alone.

Little did we know when we first started that all this was subtle preparation for a far greater tragedy that was still on the horizon: the pandemic of AIDS. It took twenty years for the American people to feel more comfortable talking about death, openly discussing the possible use of a hospice and/or palliative care unit for elderly parents. Now, millions of young people are faced with premature death, and the number of hospice and hospital beds available to them is far too small to accommodate their needs.

Not only do people with AIDS have to go through the "stages of dying," they are faced with issues the world never has had to deal with to such an extent, in such massive numbers, and from every direction. AIDS has become our largest sociopolitical issue, a dividing line of

4

religious groups, a battleground for ambitious medical researchers, and the biggest demonstration of man's inhumanity to man—even far exceeding the treatment of leprosy patients in Damien's days.

When AIDS started to appear in the United States in the late seventies, no one in the government, or in the medical profession, had any idea the extent to which this soon-to-become epidemic disease would alter the life and life-expectancy of thousands (if not millions) of people the world over. Tragically, the "stages of dying" are experienced by millions in America today. Feelings of denial abound when it comes to facing the reality of a son's homosexuality; a child's contact and infection with the AIDS virus; a husband's bisexuality that led to an infected newborn baby. And when it comes to being more careful about any sexual encounter or the use of needles for illegal drugs, thousands more still live with the illusion that it cannot happen to them.

Denial is a difficult defense and it cannot be maintained over a long period of time unless parents totally avoid contact with their children and "keep their heads in the sand." Just as Americans have been known to be a death-denying people, so it has become quite obvious that we also attempt to deny AIDS, to pretend it is none of our business! We hear weekly, from thousands of pulpits, "love thy neighbor," but when it comes to putting that into practice we quickly add a few conditions. And it is those who preach the loudest who have shown the poorest records in their care and compassion.

When a mother discovers that the cause of her baby's AIDS is her husband of ten years, she desperately tries to deny the possibility that he has a history of bisexual behavior. Even if he eventually admits it, she still tries to find another reason for the infection. One such woman even accused her pediatrician of having used unclean needles on her infant son despite the fact that her husband proved to be an AIDS carrier and admitted to having had a long-standing affair with one of his male co-workers.

Once families can no longer maintain denial, anger and rage set in. A German family was so upset and furious when the casket containing their son was shipped to their hometown marked in big letters "AIDS," that they left— never to return—the village where the family had lived for several generations.

Fury and anger is obvious in the "solutions" so many apparently well-meaning citizens present in their orato-ries and offer to "put all AIDS carriers on an island, or in some sort of camp where they can be watched and unable to spread the dreaded disease." Does that sound a bit like Molokai in the last century or the Nazi concentration camps, where they "isolated" the unwanted race or all those who did not agree with the Führer? We have in-deed learned very little from history.

Does it remind you a bit of the war in Vietnam, where we were exposed daily to such statements as "Ten Vietcong were killed, but only one American." Yes, we still live in the illusion that it shall happen to thee and thee, but not to me. How many more wars, epidemics, famines, or other tragedies do we humans need before we open our minds, hearts, and ears and finally believe that whatever happens to our fellow man happens to us? We were taught that we are our brother's keeper, but we quickly add all sorts of conditions before we even consider such a possibility.

Anger comes in many forms with the AIDS epidemic. When I called the higher authorities of our penal system

6

years ago to offer a plan as to how to avoid the spreading of AIDS in our prisons, I was told, "This problem simply does not exist." They assured me that they had had only four such patients in the system, and three of them had already been released! The following day I visited a prison that had *seven* AIDS patients housed in one wing. No, denial will not work, and anger at the sick men and women will help neither those afflicted nor those who don't know how to cope with the ever-increasing reality that this is an illness that will continue to spread until we learn to change our ways!

I became very angry myself when one of the bedridden inmates I had visited asked for some oatmeal or anything that he still might be able to swallow—and they brought him tacos! This man was literally starving to death because he had a fulminating infection in his mouth and throat and was unable to receive adequate soft foods, which might have at least made him a little more comfortable. A transfer to a city hospital was out of the question because it would take too much time to handle the red tape. It is this disguised anger, this passive-aggressive hostility that was rampant in the early years of AIDS in the United States—not only in the penal system but everywhere in our communities.

With a sweet smile on his face, a minister informed one of my female AIDS patients that she was no longer able to attend Sunday services as her presence would empty the church rapidly and he did not like preaching to empty pews! The same thing happened to the unmarried mother of a dying three-year-old when she needed the support of her church more than ever.

How many children who had attended Sunday school for years were confused by the dichotomy between what they were taught and what they witnessed when an infected hemophiliac was refused permission to attend school. The anger, frustration, and toll on energy parents feel is often insurmountable when it comes to standing up to the community or school board. And since this happens when the family is already suffering sleepless nights—from worries about the next ominous symptom of their child, from concerns over the ever-increasing cost of tests and available treatments—there is little if any energy left "to fight city hall." They either give up or withdraw from the community to live out the last few weeks or months together in as peaceful an environment as they are able to muster. And again, it becomes evident that those who stick together will be strengthened, and those who have to struggle alone either fall apart or withdraw completely, abandoning a baby in the hospital in order to "disappear from society." At least this way they know their child has good medical and nursing care and they can go someplace where no one knows them and quietly die in a rented apartment or room.

"Bargaining" is evident in older children and adults, as well as in the family, and often in the health-care providers: "If she only makes it to first grade, then her immune system will be stronger and she can lick this disease." One prostitute said to me, "If my child gets well, I promise I will live like a nun thereafter." It was not to be: both died within seven months of each other. Then there are the mothers who, upon hearing of their sons' AIDS, move clear across the country, strongly believing that if they give up their homes and work to care for their "boys," their sons will make it.

Naturally, depending on the course of the illness, this type of thinking does not stand up very long. It is gradu-

8

ally replaced with a mixture of anger, frustration, exhaustion, and *depression*. Different from patients with cancer, or other more "acceptable" illnesses, this depression cannot be shared with many. The man whose wife has cancer finds compassion, a listening ear, organizations: clergy, hospital personnel, relatives, and friends who will pitch in and listen to his grieving for hours. They can empathize with the man who has to hold down a job, then come home and cook dinner, who has to learn to do the shopping and laundry, and get the children to bed and to school early the next morning.

Yet if this man's wife was suffering from AIDS, he'd see little of his neighbors, and if they occasionally did some shopping for him, they'd drop the groceries in front of the apartment door with the excuse, "I did not want to disturb you."

Someone whose next of kin is dying of AIDS may desperately need to lean his head on a shoulder, but he will not even get as much as a handshake out of fear that the disease can be spread this way. The barbershop—often a place where people can pour out their hearts—may be closed to him with the explanation that the barber had to cut down his clientele and is no longer available to give him his regular haircuts. The same treatment may await him at the dentist's office, or in the neighborhood bar, where his old buddy suddenly has an important appointment and leaves in a rush when he shows up. One formerly very uptight couple became so frustrated when a well-known Californian funeral chain refused to bury their son that they sought help in the gay community, which had buried hundreds of their own friends. Those men not only welcomed the couple warmheartedly, but arranged the whole funeral and attended in great numbers to show that not everybody in the world had forgotten and forsaken them! They sobbed and cried at the funeral not only because of their sadness over the death of a young, talented, promising son, but also out of gratitude that this tragic illness truly separated the wheat from the chaff.

Depression is evidenced among the gay population, who attend the funerals of more young men cut down in the prime of their lives than one could ever think possible. One of my patients said sadly that it might be a blessing that he had become bedridden; going to funerals every single week had begun to wear him down emotionally and physically.

No, nobody affected by this illness ever gets used to the absenteeism among colleagues and friends, and then, too, the ever smaller number of healthy friends. Even a slight cold in the winter is viewed as an ominous sign, and every cough is believed to be the beginning of pneumonia as a result of AIDS. A patient of mine who suddenly showed bloody spots on his skin was convinced that he was "the next victim" (his own phrase), and was surprised and "almost happy" when the diagnosis turned out to be leukemia. He struggled with leukemia for a couple of years before he died, and pathetically said that he did not even dare to become depressed about his poor prognosis; he was just so happy he did not have AIDS!

Will AIDS patients ever reach a stage of acceptance and peace? Yes, the same is true as with all other terminally ill patients. If they receive and give themselves enough permission to express their anguish and their tears, their sense of impotence against a vicious killer virus and against a society that discriminates, judges, blames, and viciously enjoys the "fruit of these patients' unhealthy life-styles"; if they have enough of a support system with people who simply love and accept them and give them the natural nurturing that all human beings need, especially when they are sick, then, and then only, will they develop the stage of peace and serenity that makes the transition we call death a quiet slipping over into another form of existence.

Yes, there are many who do not receive this kind of help. There are many who are judged and discriminated against to the end. There are many who are shipped around and have no one with whom to share their pain. The human spirit, however, is strong, and I have seen the hardest inmates become soft and forgiving to those who purposely made their last months miserable beyond comprehension. In those last few weeks or days, many of them had visions, became aware of help from beyond. And some of them wrote the most profound letters—letters that should make us ashamed in the face of such genuine spirituality.

Yet of all the thousands of patients I have seen literally all over the world, I have never seen such mutual support and solidarity as I have among AIDS patients themselves and their partners. Young men risked their lives in the early days of the epidemic when we were quite ignorant about the transmission of the disease. They were willing to hold those young dying men in their arms so they would not feel unloved and deserted at the end of their lives. In those days they were unaware that one could not catch the disease by sheer proximity, yet they were still willing to risk their young lives to ease their friends' suffering.

I believe that in view of man's horrible history of destructiveness toward the world of nature, man against man, we have been given many chances to learn our lessons. And there were many great teachers who attempted to prepare us. But we, in our own arrogant, grandiose ways, thought we knew better—for ourselves and for our country. We gradually replaced the old inner knowledge of our spiritual origin with the "god of material wealth and power, politics, and conditional love." We learned very little from the world wars, from Korea, Vietnam, Biafra, Beirut, Ireland, Ethiopia . . . to name just a few of the tests we were given. One war escalated into another, one religion fought against the other—in the name of God! We were always able to turn off the radio or the TV if it started to get to us, and so we needed a reminder that we could not continue our destructiveness against nature and against our fellow man any longer—or else there would be no planet Earth left.

Is it possible that our AIDS patients, children and adults alike, chose to contribute their short life spans on planet Earth to help us open our eyes, to raise our consciousness, to open our hearts and minds, and to finally see the light?

This is what I see as the often predicted separation of the wheat from the chaff, which is meant to happen before the second coming. We can destroy ourselves with our own self-imposed fears, blame, shame, negativity. We can become very vulnerable to diseases, and more panicky when the number of AIDS patients reaches a million and more. Or we can make our choices based on love and begin to heal, to serve those with AIDS and other diseases, to show compassion and understanding, and finally, before it is too late, to learn the final lesson, the lesson of unconditional love.

12

Over the next ten years, as changes take place on Earth, those who choose love *now* will have nothing to fear. They will be spiritually uplifted and above all the turmoil. Those who stick to their old negative, judgmental ways will blame everybody and everything and will be too blind to see the destiny they have created for themselves.

Since we can no longer deny that AIDS is a life-threatening illness that will eventually involve millions of people and decimate large portions of our human population, it is our choice to grow and learn from it, to either help the people with this dread disease or abandon them. It is our choice to live up to this ultimate challenge or to perish.

Chapter 1

Working with AIDS Patients

My work with AIDS patients started right at the beginning of the epidemic, totally unplanned and spontaneous, as all my work had proceeded in the previous two decades, if it were not already my whole life-style! In the early eighties, we knew very little about this peculiar disease. All we heard (and mainly from the West Coast gay community) was that new cases were diagnosed daily and that many of those young men were dying rather rapidly. There were no cases of homosexual women reported to have contracted the disease. No one knew much about the mode of transmission. The general public just started to become afraid of the upcoming news on radio and TV, but did not feel threatened because "it happened to others," people with whom they felt they had "very little in common anyway," as a former neighbor expressed it.

It all began early in 1981 when I received a phone call from a stranger who asked rather shyly if I would consider taking an AIDS patient to one of my five-day workshops. He seemed to doubt that he'd get an affirmative answer. "Naturally," I said. "We have never ever discriminated, and all terminally ill patients have always been welcome." We view these workshops as their last chance to put "their houses in order," to finish their "unfinished business," and to make peace with whomever they still had disagreements. We are also proud of our well-received pain management for dying patients, and we pride ourselves on the fact that most of our cancer patients die fully conscious and in peace, most often at home rather than in an institution. After I hung up, I started to think, "What if the other hundred participants in the workshop do not agree with my decision and simply take off? What if they refuse to talk to him? To eat at the same table? There were a thousand questions. Did we need to have special eating utensils for him, or was it established that the disease was not contagious? Should we notify the workshop site to have a separate set of bedsheets, and to separate the laundry? God, there were so many things to consider and so little time left. I was glad, however, for the patient's initiative. He was obviously highly motivated and would surely "push many buttons" for the other participants, who could only benefit from his presence.

On a Monday, at noon, all 101 people showed up at the retreat. We shared our first lunch together in order to slowly get acquainted. Since I have no memory for names, I did not pay much attention when Bob introduced himself to me. I did not associate the person with the earlier phone call. What impressed me, however, in a rather shocking and, for me, unexpected manner, was his face. His nose was huge and purple. His face, neck, and arms

15

were covered with purplish patches, which would later in the decade become synonymous with Kaposi's sarcoma, one of the most dreaded malignancies and often associated with AIDS. His visual appearance was almost repulsive at first. Being a physician, I was used to all sorts of horrible sights, both from working in the Dermatologic Hospital in Zurich with patients who had venereal disease (prior to penicillin!), and later on, in emergency rooms. I could not help, however, watching the faces of the less indoctrinated workshop participants, who most likely had never been in the company of such a person.

What occurred over the next few days would not only be an incredible lesson for me, but it set the tone for all our forthcoming workshops in the United States, Europe, Canada, New Zealand, and Australia. By Tuesday evening, after our AIDS patient had shared every meal so far sitting next to me, I noticed that I included in my prayer: "Please, Lord, let me have one single meal in an appetizing environment." I jolted up in an instant! Did I, Elisabeth, really say that in a prayer to the Lord, who was known to work with the lepers and who tried to set an example for all of us to share, to love, to heal? I have never in my life worked harder to get in touch with my own feelings of repulsion, my own concerns, my shame and guilt than I had that night! Thank God for my assistants, who were there when my physical stamina started to wear out from paying attention to 101 people for five days and five nights.

When Bob began to feel comfortable and started to share the nightmare of being a twenty-seven-year-old man who got sicker and sicker every week without knowing the cause of all these infections, everybody sat and listened to him. It was upon reading an obituary in a gay

16

newspaper that it hit him like lightning that he, too, could be a victim of this still-quite-unknown disease. His illness progressed with unusual rapidity, but he, fortunately, had a friend who did the shopping for him—and not just the shopping for the daily food, but also for more information. To the growing pile of pamphlets on his table were added every news clipping—at a time when the news media regarded this new disease as a real "hot item." He went from shock to denial, from anger and rage to bargaining with God. There were days when he was so depressed he could neither eat nor sleep. The sores in his mouth and throat added to his discomfort. He blamed his inability to swallow as the cause of his extraordinary weight loss. He avoided his family out of fear of their reaction and started to isolate himself totally.

What were once pleasures became sad reminders of what his life was like "before." One day, he recalled, his mother called from out of state, and before he could say "hello," she questioned him in an almost accusing way, "You are not gay, are you?" Later he recalled that he was grateful for her initiative. He blurted out, "Yes, Mom, I am." Nothing more was said, and he knew that she might have suspected (initiated by all the newspaper information) that he was really sick and might have this dreaded disease. Bob then started to cry like a baby. He held his pillow in his arms, sobbing into it, again and again repeating, "I'm sorry, Mom, I'm sorry."

There were very few dry eyes in the room. Two other mothers who suspected their sons to be gay and possible candidates for AIDS cried openly. Both of them left the workshop with an increased understanding and compassion. They both visited their sons to share their experience with the workshop and Bob, and later became a

17

great support system for their sons when they became confirmed AIDS patients.

Bob spent many more sessions of sharing, both in the large room and in a more private separate room, to finish his unfinished business. Even the most judgmental ministers had tears in their eyes and approached him with a big hug! The ice was broken! Instead of judgment and more guilt, they grew in true understanding and compassion. I was not surprised when all 101 people lifted Bob up at the end of the evening session and, while gently rocking him, sang "I'll be loving you, always."

Privately I thanked God that night for giving me intuition and making a spontaneous choice from my spiritual quadrant and not from my head. Had I made my choice to take or reject him from my intellect, I might have waited and it could have been too late for Bob and the many others who followed him. The moment I could see him as a suffering human being with incredible inner beauty and honesty, I no longer had any problems either sharing meals or hugs with him. And, as is so often the case, the group took the cue from their leader and followed. It was a profound, though painful, experience that would have many ramifications in the years to come.

When Bob died he was surrounded not only by his family, but also by many of the new friends he made at the workshop. He was wearing one of my scarfs, which has become such an important part of our workshops. Since we have had an ever-increasing number of patients (cancer, multiple sclerosis, lupus, AIDS patients) who are unable to pay for the five-day workshops, I started to knit scarves during my many hours of flying from continent to continent (no two are alike and their colors, naturally, have great significance). At the end of a five-day workshop

18

we hold a raffle and auction, and some very wealthy people pay horrendously large sums for these scarves with the label, "Hand made by EKR." (Very often, this treasure would be passed on to a patient who wore it at the time of death, often leaving a note to pass it on to another patient.) The money earned from those scarfs have paid for all our indigent patients for the past eight years; we have never had to turn any needy patient down because we have this "Scholarship Fund," as we lovingly call it.

A workshop with only AIDS patients was the next logical step as the number of requests from these patients far exceeded the places we had available, and we were always booked six to twelve months ahead of time. When an AIDS patient called we could not allow him to wait that long; we had no guarantee that he would still be alive in a year. Thanks to Hal Frank from San Diego, who used to work in my office, a place was found in northern California where AIDS patients were welcome. The retreat was in an isolated but absolutely gorgeous setting, the food healthy, and the atmosphere one of love and mutual trust.

I shall never forget the time spent up there. By then I was not living in California any more and no longer exposed to many AIDS patients, so I was still shocked at the physical appearance of these young men. They were all between twenty-one and thirty-nine years of age, all of them were sick, many of them dying. Some were so weak they had to lie on the floor during the whole session. I have never in my life seen so much genuine caring and sharing, loving and holding, as I saw during that workshop! The volunteers who assisted were the warmest, most caring women and men I have ever met and would,

19

in years to come, make headlines and set up programs for psychological and physical support of these patients.

The stories of the AIDS patients almost repeated themselves. First, they had to come to grips with telling their families that they were homosexuals. They could not postpone that fact much longer since they had more and more hospitalizations, and sooner or later the families would know anyway. The reactions of the next of kin were manifold: from shock and total rejection to loving and supportive care. Mothers, although more dismayed about those facts, did come to their sons' help more often than fathers, who regarded them as "not worthwhile being called my son," or simply and silently "had nothing to do with them."

After sharing the reaction of the next of kin, which usually was the first and hardest lesson many of them had to learn, the reaction of society at large came up: the dentist who "refused to fix his teeth"; the cab drivers who refused to take them to the hospital when they were in dire need of emergency treatment. Many health-care professionals themselves treated the AIDS patients worse than leprosy patients, often keeping them waiting for hours or until they passed out in a little side room, where they had been placed and then "forgotten." They would wear masks and gowns just to talk to them or they would sit five feet away from them while getting information. When one of the patients wanted to make a phone call, the nurse screamed at him, "Don't you touch that phone," and then scrubbed it as if he had vomited on it. So many insults, so many rejections, so many painful memories. There were lovers who decided to kill their friends and then commit suicide since "they were going to die anyway." The issue of passive and active euthanasia was coming up again and again. It was the time when San Francisco just started organizing support systems, a special unit for these patients, and a hot line for questions, loneliness, isolation, and, naturally, emergencies.

A bisexual man was present who discussed his horrible guilt and inability to share his thoughts with his wife, who had just given birth to a baby with AIDS. He actually envied many of the men who had male mates with whom they were able to share their problems, dilemma, and grief. He was tempted to leave his family altogether, but was unable to do so because of the sick baby, for whom he took the entire blame. During these very painful and "heavy" days, there was one man who just beamed during the whole session. I was tempted to holler at him, "What's the matter with you, are you sick?" But I restrained myself. Just a short while before the end of the workshop and my departure, I confronted him in as much of an unjudgmental manner as I was able to muster. "I noticed that you smiled the whole day; what caused this unusual reaction?" I asked him. His smile grew wider. "Yes," he said, "I'm glad you asked. If I may, I would like to share with the group why this illness has become my biggest blessing." He then proceeded to share his early childhood in a very fundamental Christian family of the South. He realized as a young teenager that he was homosexual. He tried to hide it from his family but was unable to do so. Sessions with his pastor and their church group only made his feelings of total rejection and guilt worse. He was now ostracized by the whole community. The tension grew at home, no one was willing to talk to him. The father tried to curtail his activities and forced him to work at the family business so he could keep an eye on him every minute of the day.

When he left for the West Coast, he was determined never to walk into that home again, never to talk to his parents again. His life in the "big city," although exciting at first, was not what he had hoped for. He never found the right job, and once he started to make friends he got introduced into a life-style that was very different from what he imagined his life would be.

Years passed and he found himself dying in the AIDS ward of the city hospital. He had just gone through weeks of agonizing pain, diarrhea, and vomiting. He was emaciated beyond recognition. There were only two friends left who continued to visit him; more than two dozen of his former friends had preceded him in death. He did what most of us will do in moments like this: He reviewed the windstorms of his life, of which there were many. It is true they had made him strong, self-sufficient, and independent, but it had been a short and most painful life. And then he started to drift off into a half sleep and began to review what we call the "moments." Moments are those, often too few, instances where someone in our life shows us true love. When someone just takes us in his or her arms and hugs us without an explanation. When someone (usually a grandmother or grandfather) shows that he cares—not because of our achievements, but just because of us.

All the moments he could recall were linked with his father and his mother. How are they now? Have they aged? Were they worried? Were they well? A million questions came to his mind. He knew he really looked horrible, but he needed to see them once more before he died. He needed to tell them of his discovery that his special moments were all connected with them. The time was running out and he did not want to die without one more hug and thank-you. His doctor understood his plight. He called his mother up. She had the same voice. She did not even seem too surprised to hear from him after so many years of silence. She was very loving and straightforward, "We are looking forward to seeing you once more, son." After she hung up, he cried. He had to admit to himself that he had told her a half-lie. He told her that he was dying of cancer and wanted to see her once more. He was surprised how calmly she took the news. But he really did not want to think too much about the "once" more.

He needed to get strong enough to make the trip. He needed to borrow money for the flight. He needed a haircut and someone to shave him, and that would be a problem because of the many lesions on his face. The big day arrived. He had to borrow a suit from one of his friends, since all his clothes were far too big on him. He looked once more in the mirror. God, how long had it been since he looked at himself as an outsider would see him. He looked very emaciated, very clean . . . but he was on his way home! He then recounted how he crossed the meadow, approaching the log house in which he had spent his childhood. The dog came running like an old friend. Nothing seemed to have changed. His mother was sitting on the front porch and his father was sitting in a rocking chair, reading the newspaper. Mom held both arms up as she ran toward him, and Dad followed somewhat slower behind her. (They're always a little behind.) A few feet short of their meeting, a thought came to his mind that almost made him stop. God, what would happen if she really saw the purple lesions on his face? If she would stop and hesitate? If she would put her arms down and stop a few feet before they would hug each other?

23

His heart was racing, his feet were barely able to carry him by now. Yes, this trip was probably more than his body could take. The last thought he could remember was, "I have to face this as just another challenge and not a threat." Then he was in his mother's arms. She had not stopped. She had not hesitated. They both had their arms around each other. Then he heard his mother's voice whispering in his ear, "Son, we know you have AIDS and it's okay with us."

Their tears mingled and no other words were necessary. "You see," our friend said, "I had to have this dreadful disease to learn, to really know what unconditional love is all about." This story was the climax of our workshop. It gave hope to all those who had experienced so much rejection in their all-too-short lives. It gave awareness to all of us about the essentials in life, the true sharing and acceptance of another human being—regardless of color, creed, or sexual preference. And for this, I say, "The AIDS epidemic will turn out to be the biggest and best teacher."

Let us visit some other AIDS patients and see how the disease has changed their lives. Mr. and Mrs. S. have only been married two years. They were looking forward to the birth of their first child, and when Suzie was born she appeared sickly almost from the beginning. The young mother also started to have spells of extreme fatigue, night sweats, and a general malaise, all of which were attributed to a young mother who had just given birth to her first child.

But life, instead of being exciting and happy, became almost a burden. Mother and child appeared to be sick, and getting sicker. The young father worried, spent seemingly endless days in doctors' offices and outpatient clinics, and received little advice or help. No one seemed to know what was wrong with the mother, or the little baby who just did not seem to thrive.

It was five months later that a new physician was consulted and diagnosed AIDS in both the mother and child. By then, the married life of the couple had practically ceased. The father was barely able to hold onto his job, and the bills were piling up. There was no laughter or singing in the house anymore, and it seemed that everyone concerned was living in a morgue. The days were spent in a hospital room looking out onto the brick wall of another building or staring into space. The conversation was sparse and the interaction between the couple was practically nil.

How does a young couple deal with such a tragedy? The father's concern was focused on the ability or inability to keep his job. Can he tell his boss and co-workers that both his young wife and his first and only child are dying of this dread disease? Is he going to be fired, or shunned by his colleagues? Are they going to move away when he wants to join them in the cafeteria? Are they going to be afraid that he may have caught the disease since he had a regular intimate relationship with his wife when she was already sick but undiagnosed? Is he going to have to see his wife die before the baby? How is his family going to react to all of this? Is the life insurance he had on his wife going to be canceled because she had AIDS, the "forbidden disease"? There were so many questions that went through his mind and so few people with whom he was able to discuss them. He felt as if he was living through a nightmare, but he realized there would be no awakening, and no resumption of the marriage that he had planned so very, very differently just a couple of years ago. What made it more difficult was the fact that it was determined that she contracted theAIDS virus two years prior to their marriage as a result of a blood transfusion that was almost certainly an unnecessary procedure as a result of dental surgery. But there was no use thinking backward. It was all very depressing. He looked at his young wife, who had aged a lot in the past few months. She just sat there holding the quiet baby in her arms, not talking to her or to him. Sometimes he wished they would just share what was going on inside their minds, but neither one wanted to hurt the other, and the result was a silent communion between the three who shared the same tragic destiny that was really beyond comprehension. Where is the support system for such families? There are many groups to help the thousands of gay men who have been affected by this disease, but too few who are familiar and ready to pitch in and help the stricken average, middle-class families who are totally unprepared for such a tragedy and who often remain in an almost permanent state of shock from which the surviving spouse "wakes up" only after the mate and child are buried. What are the chances of starting from scratch again? What woman would have the courage to marry a man after he lived for a couple of years with a wife who died of AIDS?

Mrs. P. was a woman who tried to raise her three-year-old son, John, by herself in a small Virginian community. She made a marginal living and managed quite well as long as John was well. But for the last year he had been sickly, and she finally had to give up her job to take care of his recurrent colds, pneumonias, and diarrhea. One illness led to the other, she had many doctors and a dozen diagnoses for her little one. The table in her small bedroom was covered with medicines, all of which were supposed to treat symptoms and, hopefully, make him well. Now he was slowly dying; he was no longer crying, nor was he moving around. He was just sitting in the big armchair, his eyes half-closed, and he hardly touched any food or liquid. No, she did not want to leave him in a hospital, alone again. She knew that he would die soon, and she would be left alone in this world. Life had not been easy, but somehow she would survive. She would probably move away, to someplace where nobody knew her, and nobody would ask any questions. She was sorry that she never asked anybody to take a picture of her little boy when he was well and laughing so that she could carry his photograph with her wherever she went. She could not go to her pastor, or to the local church, because they told her that AIDS was a punishment from God and all the people "like her" were of Satan and deserved what was coming to them. None of the neighbors knew of her problems except that her child was sick most of the time. God, how she would appreciate it if just one person would knock at the door and bring her a home-cooked meal, something she had not had since her little boy had stopped eating! She continued to daydream about a family who would support her, about her mother, who, instead of sitting around drunk almost all the time, would visit her grandson and take him for a ride in the stroller since he could no longer walk! Where were all the good Christian ladies and the neighborly love that she had heard about in Sunday school? Did they exist somewhere; was she simply in the wrong place?

Chapter 2

Parents of Children with AIDS

What can those of us who do not have AIDS, but have children, learn from all of this? Maybe the most important lesson is to be open and honest with each other, with every member of our family, to allow each to share whatever occupies his or her mind from the very beginning, be it husband and wife or parent and child. As long as a door is open for communication, the chances are small that this door will ever be totally and completely closed, especially during a life-threatening illness or the impending death of a member of the younger generation.

In the coming years, it will be the younger generation that will have to deal with this illness. They will no longer be able to say, "It is a gay disease, we have nothing to do with it." They will no longer be able to say that this will only happen in New York or San Francisco, because 80 percent of the future cases are projected to happen elsewhere, with an ever-increasing number of heterosexuals involved, and many more women and children. It will become the number one concern for teenagers and adolescents who will no longer be able to have sexual partners as their parents' generation did, who will no longer be able to have several intimate relationships before they decide on a partner for life. In fact, they may, literally, have to choose a celibate life if they want to be sure not to get AIDS. Whole sexual life-styles have changed already in the United States and abroad, and will change much more drastically when it becomes widely known that this disease can be transmitted through any—even regular—sexual intercourse since no one really ever knows another person's past sexual or drug history. No one will ever again be sure that the partner has not had a bisexual affair or experimented with drugs at one time or another. Perhaps one especially drastic example of this was Ms. G., a successful executive in a well-known international, highly competitive business. She had led a rather sheltered life, she never used drugs and drank very little alcohol even during the very frequent conventions, where she was mainly in the minority, as few women had yet gained so high a level of executive status. She was much sought after by colleagues who admired her business success while maintaining her femininity. She spent most of her life attending courses to establish herself as an expert, and played tennis and jogged to keep herself fit and in superior physical condition.

In a rare weak moment during one of these conventions in Atlanta, she fell head over heels in love with one of the attending chief executives. They spent a night together and never saw each other again—Mr. X. was married and worried that this "sidestep" could become public and jeopardize his business position and long-standing marriage. At that time, no one knew anything about his private life, which he had kept strictly secret. It was only after Ms. G. suddenly became very ill and was diagnosed with AIDS that a search for the origin of her infection led straight to her one-night lover whose business meetings apparently always involved visits to prostitutes!

Ms. G. killed herself with an overdose of sleeping pills. "One night of brief pleasure and this has to happen to me?!" This is an issue our generation did not have to deal with. We don't do enough to discourage young men to avoid prostitutes; we don't explain well enough to our adolescents that every partner can be a source of infection as long as he has had sexual encounters with practically anyone. We do not know who has played around with drugs, even if it was only once. We have 1.5 million to 3 million carriers of the disease, many of whom don't know they are carriers! Even though they have no symptoms and truly convince their potential bed partners that they have nothing to fear, no one is safe. Will this lead to a whole generation of celibates, of virgins—not out of any new sense of morality, but simply out of fear?

If parents again become parents (as ours were), if they take the time to listen to their children long before they are dying, and if they start early in their children's pre-teen years to openly and unashamedly talk about sexuality, much heartache could be avoided. If the parents of any of our earliest AIDS patients had done so and understood that their children were homosexuals, not sinners nor "of satan," but simply people whose sexual preference was not of the majority, many would have been able to stay in monogamous relationships and, perhaps, not had so many partners—and not spread this epidemic in such a rampant fashion.

Had they listened early to their children, they may have been able to understand why they were tempted to try drugs; they may have been able to talk with them about the dangers of drugs and kept them interested in less risky adventures. And so, what we are learning now from all the mistakes of a very busy, materialistic generation of all too busy parents is to worry less about what college their child will attend one day, but to keep the doors of understanding, mutual respect, and unconditional love open and to educate themselves and their children about issues we are too bashful to talk about until it is too late. Instead of worrying that free needle distribution to already known drug addicts would be too costly, we need to figure out where the millions of dollars will come from when we are faced with 250,000 new AIDS patients before the turn of the century.

If we, as parents, are concerned about what the neighbors may think should they find out that our son is a homosexual, we had better wonder how *we* would deal with the knowledge that he has died of AIDS!

What this epidemic teaches us is to become honest again, to talk and listen to each other, to accept and love each other more, and, most important, to learn to get our priorities straight.

Since I have worked with so many AIDS patients, who usually have a shorter life expectancy after diagnosis than most of my patients with cancer, multiple sclerosis, etcetera, I am impressed by how much faster people can come to grips with these issues and the little time they require "to see the light." Parents who never told a child that he was loved make the most heartfelt confession at the side of a son dying with AIDS. "They grow by leaps and bounds" as someone told me who shared the same experiences with formerly very reserved and "straight" parents who were experts in criticizing. Yet the question remains, "Why do we need such a harsh teacher?"

While many of the parents of my AIDS patients have done a relatively poor job in sex education and shown little understanding for their youngsters, who grew up in the promiscuous sixties, many of them rallied to their sons when it became evident that they suffered from AIDS and were in need of help.

When I make house calls to AIDS patients, I'm always struck by how many mothers really play the heroic role. Being mostly in their fifties and sixties and looking forward to an easy retirement, not only were so many expectations shattered, but many of them had to give up their professions and regular incomes as well as the place they called home and expected to spend their old age. In addition, they had to "train themselves to be moms again for little, helpless children" in a grown-up body, as one mother so aptly put it.

This woman learned of her son's illness in the fall a couple of years ago and, after a telephone conversation with him, sensed that he was much sicker than she expected. After a sleepless night she decided to head East to see for herself. She sold her home, gave up her job, and is—at the time of this writing—still sharing a small apartment in New York with her presently dying son. What used to be a healthy, strong, good-looking, and professionally well-to-do young man, the pride of her family, is now a shadow figure of a man whose age is undefinable. Like so many of these patients, he has aged an awful lot in the two and a half years he has been sick. He can no longer

32

wear any of his clothes; they "hang on his bones, fit for a halloween party," she said with dry humor.

She carries him in her arms to the bathtub—an exhausting job—and literally diapers him so she doesn't have an enormous amount of wash day after day. When he is clean and dry and smells good, she sits back with exhaustion only to repeat the whole procedure an hour later, when the bed is soiled again and he is covered with sweat.

"The nights are the most exhausting times of my life," she said with a sigh. "When he moans and groans all night long and sometimes he screams in pain." Naturally, like all mothers, she cannot understand why the doctors won't give him enough pain medication to allow him a few hours of sleep. When asked if that was for her or for her son, she resolutely said, "You bet we both need it!" Each one wants to allow the other to sleep, but while the son is unaware of his constant moaning and groaning, the mother is afraid to crawl over to his side of the room out of fear of waking him from the few moments of rest he has had all night.

Her only reprieve is the few hours she is permitted to leave the flat, to go shopping or to catch some fresh air. She depends on her son's friends—all homosexuals—upon whom she would have frowned a few years earlier. Now "they are her friends and her salvation," and she has grown and learned more in the last two years than all the earlier years of her life. Why does it take such a tragedy to learn compassion, understanding, and love, she asks me with a boring look that required no answer—just more compassion, understanding, and love.

While I sat on the floor next to her son, holding his hand, he suddenly turned to me and asked what it was really like to die. We shared a wonderful half hour together, as I recounted my own near-death experience and the accounts of so many of my patients. The mother sat quietly next to us on a chair; then she openly and audibly said to him: "You know, I never thought that I would have to bury you. I always thought that you would look after me in my old age and in my dying. But this has been such a gift, I am forever grateful that we were able to have this special time together. I am no longer afraid of you leaving me before I rejoin you." There was the most peaceful silence in the room as we all held hands in a silent communion of people who had never known each other before.

A few hours later, after a lecture in Riverside Church, I was called by a mother with an almost identical story. I had received an emergency call with an urgent request "on short notice" to visit a son who was too sick to come to my lecture. His mother was begging me to "just add another house call if you possibly can squeeze it into your obviously busy schedule." How could I say no?

She gave me a lift through New York and led me to her small apartment where, again, the mother and the very sick son shared one room. A board divided the room to give each space to sleep on the floor, adjacent to a bathroom and kitchen. A lovely and obviously caring nurse had watched Gary while the mother brought me to their place. While she sat at the table, the mother and I sat on the floor next to the very emaciated patient, who asked me the same question the previous young man had asked. I gave him a butterfly, the symbol of our transition, and explained to him that we only leave the physical body—the soul leaves and we will be whole again after what we call death. He wanted to know all about the light we encounter, and after I answered all the questions as well as I could, I noticed that the nurse had tears in her eyes even though she had pretended not to listen to our rather intimate conversation.

While we were there, a Meals on Wheels was delivered by a young couple and I was impressed by their cheerful, caring attitude—needed more by the exhausted mother, who sleeps only a few moments every so often, than by the patient, who was unable to take more than a few swallows.

I must say that the picture of parental care has changed drastically in the last few years since we took care of our first AIDS patients. In the early eighties, this disease was viewed as a strictly gay disease and very few parents either acknowledged or were informed about a son's homosexuality; two or three years later things changed dramatically and for the better. Most parents were informed about their son's sexual preference only when the diagnosis of AIDS was made; about a third of these parents chose to no longer make that an issue and came to their child's help. Between 1984 and 1986, about half of all mothers either physically or emotionally supported their sick sons, while only a third of the fathers were able or willing to do the same.

Many of the separated or divorced mothers moved to the city in which their sick sons lived and either took turns or actively cared for the patients in a totally reversed role from their earlier relationship with their growing-up and very independent children. The many mothers I visited and supported in this tiring, exhausting, but gratifying task almost unanimously expressed the enriching aspect of this close, although unexpected, intimate relationship: "I would not have missed it for the world, although I am very sorry that his father never comes to see him." "What

I don't understand is that Gerold [ex-husband] cannot come by here once in a while. He knows his son is dying— his only son—and he does not have the nerve to face it." "Can you tell me why my husband goes on all these business trips and just calls once in a while to ask how his son is doing? He lives in the same city. He has time for all his clients, but not for his son."

Yes, compassion and understanding does not have to extend only to the sick and dying young AIDS patient, but also to his parents, especially to the father who seems to have greater difficulty accepting a homosexual son, who is then a stigma in the family when it becomes "obvious, because he is dying of AIDS." It is difficult to get into a discussion with these fathers. It is obviously too late to do anything about the sexual preference of their sons, and useless to affix blame to any one cause. Men want concrete answers, they want to know the "why" of such "an aberrant life-style and don't want to hear anything about a disease that we cannot do anything about anyway."

When I tried to turn the discussion into a "here-and-now issue," asking them if there was anything they would like to tell their sons before they died, many of them shrugged their shoulders and almost sardonically stated, "It's too late for that anyway." Some fathers, but very few, do visit the hospital during their son's last stay. However, they usually stay outside the room until someone takes them by the arm and gently shoves them next to the bed. One father said resolutely, "This is not my son, he does not look like this!" I will never forget the small voice that came out of the pillow, "Yes, Dad, it's Mike, it's me—I did lose some weight." When father and son were in each other's arms I quietly tiptoed out of the room. Mike died that night, and I know that his dad is forever grateful to the orderly who gave him a gentle kick to face his son and a final reconciliation!

Paul was a strong, healthy, well-known artist who was his father's pride and joy in the early days of his career. The photo from his marine days was on the wall and his parents tried to get him married to several of "the elite," as his mother recounted. They even dragged him to a prom where all the ladies of high society gathered and each one was prettier than the next. It dismayed his parents, and especially his grandmother, that he did not want to get engaged, and they blamed it on "the allures of a young, ambitious artist who had no time for young ladies." "Not yet," they said by way of consolation! They had no inkling, or refused to allow such a thought to cross their mind, that their son (and grandson) would never wish to marry and would never fulfill their dream of an heir to their not small family fortune. He was an only child, and they had "put all their eggs into one basket," as Paul's mother explained. They were shattered when they heard about his homosexuality. "That explains it all," said his father. They were the last words he ever uttered to his son!

Jerry had an especially difficult time during the last year and a half of his life. Although he did not have the financial difficulties so many of our patients have, he had to pay for his nursing care and tried to "buy love," which he found extremely difficult. Suddenly his disease began to affect his brain, he became very forgetful and could not remember if he had paid his bills already or if the nurse had been there or not that morning. He had trouble finding words, and more often than not was unable to make himself understood. A few weeks later his vision was almost gone and he could not recognize the few friends who continued to visit him. His mother finally placed him in an expensive nursing home "out of state," where "nobody knew that he used to be our son." He died alone, among strangers; all the money in the world did not buy the love he needed so badly.

What we have learned from all the patients we visited is that those who had a fairly average or better relationship with their parents earlier in life (before the epidemic), those who communicated on a fairly regular basis before the illness was diagnosed—even those who did it only on holidays once a year if they lived in other states—were more likely to reconverge when the crisis occurred and often brought the families together. Those who really rallied around their sick children—sons *and* daughters—were grateful for the opportunity of getting to know them better than ever before, of learning who their children really were as human beings, not as some strange aberrant person beyond the comprehension of an old-fashioned life-style that had no flexibility in it, no attempts at understanding, and certainly no compassion.

Many a mother who used to detest "faggots" found out that the very people they used to condemn were their only friends and supporters, and that without them they would not have been able to stick it out to the very end of this difficult road that these moms traveled with their dying sons.

One very indignant father with a lot of money warned his son (with whom he had very little contact in the years before his illness and premature death) not to leave any money to his gay friends or he would personally "visit and eliminate them from the planet Earth!" Yes, anger and revenge to the very end is still found among many of the fathers, maybe because their own manhood is questioned by their not having raised a son who is "a real man"—and so violence and aggression may have to be used to "prove that he is a man after all."

Chapter 3

Children and AIDS

*So long as little children are allowed to suffer, there
is no true love in this world.*

—Isadora Duncan

In a society where most people continue to consider AIDS
a "gay disease" and want nothing to do with it, it comes
as a shock to learn that little children are also being
stricken. It may even be a surprise to some that there are
still many carriers who have yet to be diagnosed and
therefore risk having terminally ill babies.

Patt Morrison of the *Los Angeles Times* wrote in July
1986:

He was weak, malnourished and ailing with pneumonia. He had been in and out of hospitals for much of
his sickly two years of life, and his medical paperwork
listed him as a possible victim of neglect. There had
even been a police protective custody hold on the
boy, and the hospital had barred his family from visiting him, since it was his family who were suspected
of neglecting him.

But it was not his family who had been slowly ruining the boy's health all those months. It was AIDS, undiagnosed for those weeks that the boy had been kept apart from the family who loved him, by people legally and morally obligated to help him.

Once AIDS was diagnosed, the boy was transferred by court order to Children's Hospital in Los Angeles, and his family was at his bedside again.

The Children's Hospital's first AIDS patient turned up in 1983. Now, having treated a good portion of young AIDS and AIDS-related complex (ARC) victims—children from San Diego to San Bernardino County, from well-to-do beach homes to impoverished barrios—the hospital has begun organizing the first AIDS pediatric unit on the West Coast, the fourth in the nation.

Such a center has, tragically, become a necessity. In a social climate where AIDS is not looked upon as just another of the illnesses "children can get," they are getting the disease—and with ever-increasing frequency.

Children born prematurely or those hurt in accidents are getting AIDS from transfusions of tainted blood, donated before screening tests were developed.

Children inherit it from a mother or father who at one time took drugs intravenously with a contaminated needle, and often the children become the second generation of AIDS victims.

One of the patients at the Children's Hospital got the virus from his mother, who died of AIDS shortly after the boy's birth; the same AIDS-tainted semen that had made it possible for her to conceive—long after the parents gave up drugs—was AIDS positive and so were they.

According to Dr. Joseph Church of the Children's

Hospital, who plans to establish the AIDS unit for children, "there have been twenty-one children so far, of an average age slightly below three years. Nine have died already. Six of the Children's Hospital cases were born prematurely and were given blood transfusions—ironically to improve their chances of survival. Five got tainted blood later in life; nine had AIDS-carrying parents, including at least two drug-using fathers who passed on the ailment to their non-drug-using wives, and a woman who had received a tainted-blood transfusion and gave birth to an AIDS-infected child, who has since died." In 1986 the Centers for Disease Control in Atlanta, Georgia, reported only 316 cases of children under age thirteen, 62 percent of whom died. Their incubation time, as well as their life expectancy, is usually shorter than that of adults. Their short lives are made up of a series of—often undiagnosed—infections, vomiting, diarrhea, and a lack of energy that should warn the pediatrician to consider the family and child's history in order to diagnose the problem early, in order to prevent such tragedies as the one described at the beginning of this chapter.

The social ostracism is perhaps as tragic to a toddler as are the frequent bouts of sickness and hospitalization. Dr. Marcy Kaplan, a social worker at Los Angeles Children's Hospital, quoted a case of a a four-year-old sufferer in central California: "A nurse there, in spite of medical privacy laws, told someone who worked with the child's father. The word spread. The father lost his job, the sick boy's siblings couldn't play with other children, and at the grocery store, the boy's mother saw aquaintances draw away from her in horror. It is a bad situation if the patients go to a clinic and if there is part-time help who find out what they have, they are treated like dirt."

Perhaps one of the most charming and adamant spokeswomen for families with AIDS babies is Helen Kushnick, who speaks publicly and has recently appeared in *U.S. News and World Report* (July 7, 1986). She and her husband, Jerold, had twins, born prematurely in 1980. Sam received contaminated blood (before it was possible to check the blood supply, which is now routinely done). After innumerable infections, much isolation, and heartaches for him, his parents, and his twin sister, he died; his twin sister remained healthy. Two years after his death the ordeal still wasn't over for his family. Sara was admitted to a public kindergarten only after a doctor was assured that she was disease free. The hardest part of the disease is fear and rejection. It is hard enough for an adult to cope with it; it's impossible to explain to a child. That's why families who have a child with AIDS go underground: "There are support groups, but with AIDS you are so alone, and so is the child."

The most publicized child case in the United States was perhaps fourteen-year-old hemophiliac Ryan White from Kokomo, Indiana. In this midwestern city north of Indianapolis, parents waged a legal battle to keep the teenager out of school. Many of these parents have since withdrawn their children from the regular school and enrolled them in the Russiaville Home Study School, which held classes in a vacant American Legion Hall. At the tender age of fourteen, this young "old" man had to learn about discrimination, fear, and hate mail—and all because he survived hemophilia and was an innocent victim of tainted blood.

Hemophiliacs are probably the highest risk group of AIDS children because they received clotting factor concentrate prior to 1985. It is estimated that 96 percent to

98 percent of all those patients have been infected, due to the fact that this blood factor is collected from thousands of donors. It is an established fact that nine thousand hemophiliacs plus an additional twenty thousand blood transfusion recipients have already been infected with the AIDS virus. The implication of this is clear: they can pass the disease on to any sexual partner (homo- or heterosexual); and they should restrain from getting married and never have children! What a destiny for any young person!

Let's talk to a mom who wants to remain anonymous and has been in hiding since her daughter died of AIDS, which she contracted as a result of life-saving procedures following a tragic accident in which A. was seriously injured.

The mother had become so paranoid and defensive that she did not even allow me to take notes or record her statements in her own words. I had to promise not to divulge her name and whereabouts before she started to open up.

She truly believes that there has been a "bad star" over her entire family for the last twenty years. Her father had health problems as long as she could remember, and her mother made ends meet by working "for rich people like a slave" in order to raise her five children. She cannot remember ever being hugged by either parent, and all the kids had to work after school as soon as they were old enough to do any kind of work. She learned to iron for the same rich family, but cannot recall if she was ever paid for it. When she was seventeen she married a man who was kind to her, and after a year her first child, a son, was born.

He had a genetic disease and died before he was two years of age. All their financial resources had been used to pay the doctor and hospital bills, and then her husband lost his job. She took on the same role she had seen her mother do for so many years. She worked hard and tried to take care of her husband and her second child, A. Ulcers and migraine headaches prevented her husband from returning to full employment, and after a few years of material hardship, "little fun and a lot of bickering," her husband was arrested for "talking back to a police officer" and was found hanged in the cell of the jail where they planned to keep him overnight. With little support and not much of a loving family left, she moved to a new location "to leave the bad life behind." They had lived there only a few months when A. was hit by a car on the way home from school. She was unconscious for several months and when she finally gained consciousness, she was severely damaged. With a lot of hard work and tenacity, mother and daughter tried to help each other and even succeeded in A.'s learning to walk and talk again.

Five years to the day after she took her first step again, A. died of AIDS. Some of the blood that she had received was contaminated. The mother's last words to me were: "Maybe it was a blessing that she was able to die. I don't know what she would have done, poor, handicapped, and perhaps unable to ever become self-supporting if I should have died before her."

Dr. Kaplan from Los Angeles states, "A number of parents we dealt with had a high level of hostility." This surprises me. Most of the parents I have talked with are beyond hostility. They are still in a state of shock and numbness, with a deep sense of incomprehensibility. They have given up making sense out of the horrors they have gone through. Many of them have lost all faith, not just in God, but in humanity as a whole. They recount some of the most inhuman treatments and remarks they have received from friends and neighbors, school officials, and, yes, church people. They ask themselves, Am I responsible for all of this? What is going to happen to my other children when they grow up and someone finds out that their brother or sister has died of AIDS? Are they going to ask if they got it through a tainted blood transfusion or are they automatically going to think that the parents were junkies or had a wild sexual life-style? Why are people so cruel to each other and to our children? What do we tell relatives about the cause of death?

One parent told of the funeral of his seven-year-old and how the funeral director refused to bury "a kid with AIDS." They had apparently called a number of funeral homes with the same result. It was the father who had the idea, fueled by his anger and resentment, to contact the gay community, who not only helped him with all the arrangements, but attended the funeral and covered the casket with flowers to pay their respects to the little girl who was shunned even after her death. "God, you know, that really changed my opinion about homosexuals," the father said. "I will never again say anything derogatory about them. I think both my wife and I would have committed suicide if it had not been for that group of young men who gave my daughter a decent funeral!"

In a society where we have lost all respect and decency in the face of such a fearful disease, is it a wonder that so many parents neither notify the authorities nor a center for disease control when they discover that their child has AIDS? Many a country doctor who has known the families all their lives, and who finally suspects AIDS in a child, will treat the infection symptomatically and write "pneumonia" on the death certificate in order to avoid the hassle and tragedy that so many of these families would otherwise have to endure on top of losing a beloved child to a prolonged and merciless illness.

Another group of children who need special consideration are adopted children. A woman who visited me prior to attending a workshop to deal with much unfinished business and guilt in connection with "having given a baby away," confessed her very promiscuous life-style with a variety of men, both heterosexual and bisexual, some of them heavy drug users. When she became pregnant she was afraid of an abortion, but even more petrified about giving birth to a baby with AIDS and being "discovered." She had never taken a blood test, also out of the fear that her way of life might become known. Rather than take any risks, she decided to forfeit all rights to the child and gave it up for adoption. She was paid the equivalent of two thousand dollars through a lawyer who dealt with "such matters" and never met the future parents of her child. Now she is haunted by a bad conscience and worries whether her child was born with this dread disease. Unable to forgive herself and having no one to talk to, she became suicidal until she attended our workshop, where she publicly confessed and was accepted as another human being. She eventually was able to learn to forgive herself.

This case reminds us, however, that potential parents of adopted children should request a blood test prior to the final adoption, and if it should be positive, they need to be informed of all the consequences and its ramifications, including the costs of caring for such a chronically ill child. Only if they are fully informed should they make the choice.

Children who have been sexually abused are also becoming a risk group. Very few people in this country are fully aware of just how many children are not only physically and emotionally but also sexually abused. If the abuser is an intravenous drug user or a bisexual man, the chances are that these children will be infected.

In our workshops, 25 percent of all participants have been sexually abused as children—from the age of a few months (used for porno films!) to the adolescent years. Much too rarely do they receive any help, and if they dare tell a mother or some significant other, they are often called liars and told to "keep their mouths shut." Needless to say, they grow into adults with very poor trust levels and even poorer interpersonal relationships. Since the law in the United States requires a parent's written consent in order to perform blood tests on a minor, it is in effect asking the abuser's permission to verify such a diagnosis. New laws for our children are mandatory in order to protect them!

In another country, a stepfather was finally "discovered" to be the abuser of a fourteen-year-old girl who was severely brain-damaged and unable to speak. He had apparently sexually misused her for years, until she was hospitalized several times and eventually diagnosed as having AIDS. Ruling out all other sources, he was finally found to be the abuser when his blood test came back positive. When he confessed, it became evident that this had been going on for many years; he had been convinced that no one would ever find out about it since "she cannot speak anyway and could never point the finger at me."

If we do not change our attitudes toward AIDS patients in general, and children specifically, we may end up with tragedies like this:

In October of 1985, a German physician put a large ad in the newspaper, pleading with a mother to return with her two-year-old daughter to his practice. The woman had brought her very frail, and obviously very sick, little girl to see the doctor and had used a wrong name for both herself and the child. The mother refused steroids or antibiotics, claiming that they lived on a biogenic farm and that other doctors had already tried to convince her to have her daughter treated that way. It was only after she left, and the results of the blood tests of both mother and child were received, that the pediatrician's suspicions were verified: They both had AIDS.

A sketch of the child was published in a widely read magazine along with a plea from the doctor. Later he was informed that this child had been brought to a nearby hospital in "sad condition," but both mother and child— using yet another name—had refused hospitalization and disappeared.

Stories like this are much more common than the medical profession or the public is aware of. As long as we discriminately ostracize the children with AIDS and their families, as long as we treat them worse than many lepers were treated, the families will prevent the sick children from receiving the help they should be getting. As long as the fathers fear losing their jobs, the mothers are stared at and not wanted in grocery stores, at school meetings or in their churches, the sick children will pay the price. And all of us are guilty as long as we pretend that it is not our business. It is your business and my business, and the sooner we plan and prepare to educate the population and help them face their fears, the better prepared we will be when this epidemic takes on bigger and more devastating proportions.

Dr. Church, from Los Angeles Children's Hospital, is convinced that the number of little children who become infected through their infected parents will grow. And many of these parents show the same reactions as parents who have just been told that their child has a malignancy. No one expects children to die of cancer until it hits your own family. The difference with children who suffer from AIDS is that the parents don't know what to tell their relatives, how to explain it to their other children if they have any. When they tell members of the family and people whom they regard as their special friends they discover rather quickly that no one wants to have much to do with them. Neighbors, formerly considered special friends, refuse to allow their children to play in the garden with the AIDS children; when the news "leaks out," which happens sometimes, the tragedy is compounded by the father's inability to hold his job; by the mother's loneliness, isolation, and increased depression; and the lack of the kind of well-organized support system available to parents of cancer children.

The law is another problem for physicians, like Dr. Church, who treat AIDS children. A pregnant woman came into the hospital with a sick child, who, it was found, suffered from AIDS. After the second child was born, the AIDS-positive mother refused to consider permanent birth control and she did not have the new baby tested for AIDS. California AIDS laws were not written with children in mind! Under the law, and under penalty of a $10,000 fine and jail time, an AIDS blood test cannot be given without the written informed consent of the subject, which, in case of children, means youngsters from a few months old cannot be tested! Assemblyman Art Agnos of San Francisco has drafted a "clean-up" bill to give doctors easier access to test results. It would give guardians the right to consent to blood tests for minors, and allow involuntary blood testing for convicted rapists or high risk foster children before placing them in foster homes.

Chapter 4

Babies with AIDS: We the People

Dear Dr. Kübler-Ross,

I am writing to you on the evening of November 16, 1985, in a small town in northern New Hampshire, as the first snow of the season falls outside. I feel compelled to write to you about my daughter, who died one and a half months ago of AIDS. She was only nine months old.

I am not sure what it is that I want to write here . . . maybe I am trying to rid myself of grief and frustration, and although I have never met you, I know how closely you live with death, and I'm familiar with your tremendous compassion and humanitarism toward the sick and dying. I have also been told, from a social worker, Maris N., at the local hospital, that you are in the process of organizing a hospice that deals specifically for children with AIDS. As I am sure that you know, this is a truly dreadful disease, and it's agony to watch anyone dwindle away at the mercy of it, let alone a child. Losing my daughter was the most devastating experience of my life, but once I had accepted the fact that her chances for survival were nil, all I was really concerned about was the quality of her life during the time that she still had left. The pediatric staff, most importantly her doctor, were very understanding of this wish; G. was able to go home a few days after diagnosis, where she remained for a week or two at a time. Medical treatments were kept to a fair minimum, mostly gamma globulin treatments, antibiotics for chronic otitis media and thrush, and extra vitamin supplements. Her illness progressed swiftly, also causing atrophy of her brain and a general failure to thrive. One and a half months after diagnosis, she developed CMV pneumonia, which was the direct cause of her death one week later. I emphatically stressed that I wanted no great life-saving measures taken. Her comfort was top priority for me, and for her to be able to be home, away from the trauma of the hospital, was something I felt strongly about.

The few weeks that she did stay home, she was peaceful and generally content, with a minimum of suffering and discomfort. I will treasure that brief time, that we had together, always. I was very lucky to be able to be with G. at the hospital, when I was there, sleeping next to her in the ward at night. The nurses and interns were wonderful; extremely supportive and sensitive to my wishes for my daughter.

I want to tell you about how my baby actually died. We were alone in the hospital room, she and I, together, and I was rocking her in my arms. For the previous twenty-four hours, she had been only on morphine, with an oxygen tube in her nose to help her breathe, and everyone knew that at any time she could die. But G. kept hanging on, certainly past the time they thought she could or would, and it was agony for me, watching her struggle for her every breath. So I took her in my arms and I told her we would sit there together until she could let go. It took about half an hour, and then, finally, I felt her will leave, felt something in her stop struggling. Five minutes later she took her last breath . . . I watched her soul rise, floating toward the window on the far side of the room, and I knew my daughter was free—finally free of the pain and suffering she had endured.

I don't know why death has been taught to us as this profoundly disturbing and frightening thing, but that September evening, when G. died, it was a most natural and somehow calming process. It seemed that when I stopped resisting, and surrendered to the natural order of things, she could do the same; and sitting there, talking to her, telling her that she could let go and that there was nothing to hold on to any more, I felt I was helping her to release the life that in nine short months she had become so attached to. It was a profound revelation, having gone through the magnificant experience of her birth, helping her in her struggle to be born, and then helping her later in her struggle to die.

Of course, there is no way to escape the grief—to avoid a feeling of being robbed of a life—a life I cherished to my soul. But I know my daughter is very much alive in spirit, and I feel her all around me. It is only the body that housed her shining soul that is dead . . . and I will always feel deeply blessed at having her presence in my life, short though it was, and for all the gifts she brought to me through her being.

You can imagine I feel passionately about AIDS and I read every bit of information I can about it. I am interested now, not so much in the medical side of it, but in what kind of treatment, what kind of quality of care, what spiritual or emotional relief and comfort these people are getting. And even more importantly, are they receiving their personal and civil rights—their natural right to die with some degree of dignity and grace. I care about the horrible ostracism they experience—that "leper" brand that has been so prevalent with the "plague." I do know about this kind of isolation, as my daughter contracted AIDS from me, presumably while still a fetus. I am not sick, however, and would never even have known I was infected if not for G., and I take great pains to have this secret remain a secret. Of course, having the threat of this disease, and all its ramifications hanging over my head, is a burden. But I don't dwell on it, and I'm thankful for the continuing state of good health I find myself in.

I want to be involved with this disease, and with the people who are being touched by it, either in severe or light ways, but I am not at all sure of what I can do or what part I can play. I am single, almost twenty-three, with only a high school education to speak of. But I am deeply encouraged that you have become so involved with AIDS, and specifically with the children who are such innocent victims of it. If there is anything I can do, please write me and tell me. I feel sorry for these people, and I think, because of G., I somehow feel a responsibility; I don't want her little life or her suffering to have been in vain.

My deepest thanks and respect,
B.

Unfortunately, there are more babies like Baby G., and not all of them have the loving, caring mother she had. As more and more reports came in from other mothers with afflicted children, it became quite clear that AIDS was no longer a gay disease, but affects every age and every group.

While over the preceding years half my mail came from grieving parents and those who had little ones suffering from cancer, surprisingly the mail has shifted to mothers of AIDS babies. They were more often than not sick themselves and felt overwhelmed and at their wits' end caring for them. So many of these notes and letters were barely legible, but the utter despair they expressed, mixed with both anticipated rejection and little glimpses of hope, came through nonetheless.

Of all the notes I received during this time, the most heartbreaking was one that had been scribbled on a small piece of paper: "Dear Dr. Ross, I have a three-year-old son who has AIDS. I can no longer take care of him. He eats very little and drinks very little. How much would you charge to take care of him?"

I became increasingly involved in the plight of babies with AIDS after reading a desperate plea in a Florida newspaper. A mother was *turned down* by seventy agencies after asking for a place of care and love for her baby dying of AIDS prior to her own death. She died without ever knowing who would look after her terminally ill toddler!

My thoughts went back to three years earlier when I bought a lovely Virginian farm with the intention of having a place for rest and recuperation, to raise animals and grow vegetables, to offer my lovely land during the summer to needy inner-city children, and, hopefully, to build a center for my own workshops. I had the fantasy that this would become my *own* healing place, where I could rest between my travels and recharge my batteries so as to be better able to give to others.

But this was obviously not to be. It appeared that my work had already been cut out for me in a different direction. I had always listened to my inner guidance and I felt that I had no other choice. I had no idea what fate had in store for me—in Headwaters, Virginia, no less! But I—as I had done many times in my life—would bury my private dreams and follow my destiny.

I was soon haunted by the images of babies dying of AIDS, uncared for, in alien, institutionalized care centers instead of in a home full of love and compassion. Instead of mutual support and generous offers of help, many a family is forced to go into hiding. The most vulnerable and threatened of them all were single mothers who were former drug addicts and often terminally ill themselves. These women had previously been able to care for their children, but because of their own illness and the child's constant needs, they were unable to do so any longer. They had no support system, no church to fall back on, no husband to support them, and few if any friends left.

Hundreds of parents of hemophiliacs and other AIDS-afflicted children were faced with yet another nightmare:

their children going to school. They started to get tremendous opposition, were confronted at angry community meetings and nasty parent boycotts, as well as being flooded with hostile and threatening mail from parents of healthy children. The well-publicized family in Arcadia, Florida, whose home was burned down when the parents of the afflicted children sought legal council to permit them to attend school, is another classic case of man's inhumanity toward his fellow man.

The "threat" these small children seem to pose to their communities has brought out a level of hostility unseen in any other so-called Christian society. I watched as AIDS rapidly exploded into a major sociopolitical issue, and I vowed to help these afflicted little ones, which is when the saga began!

On June 2, 1985, I was invited to present a lecture at the Mary Baldwin College in Staunton, Virginia. As I always talk extemporaneously—I never write anything down—I felt drawn to the one issue that recently was foremost on my mind: AIDS babies and the hospice movement. The graduating class really paid attention.

Little did I know what an uproar my idea (for the first time publicly expressed) would cause! Newspaper reporters and TV people started calling and inquiring about the progress of our baby hospice, and we had to tell them that this was in the planning stages and there was no need to travel the curving country roads to come out to see us. But it was to no avail; the phones kept ringing and the uninvited visitors were adamant in coming to see our farm and our "center." In order to put a stop to the constant influx of intruders, which caused interruptions and made working very difficult, we called a news conference to take care of everybody at one time.

It turned into a pleasant day with a friendly, curious, and not-at-all hostile group of interviewers who came from all over the state, Washington, D.C., and as far away as Chicago. We promised to keep them up to date through our regular quarterly newsletter.

I spent the next several days with my farm crew, walking over my 250 acres of farmland to look for an ideal place to house the children and to erect a simple home for fifteen to twenty little toddlers and their care-givers. There was excitement and enthusiasm on the farm, far more than at any other time in the two and a half years that I had lived there. Naturally, we had a session with the staff and discussed the consequences of our choices. There was very little fear expressed and everyone had free choice to get personally involved in the care of these children or to work on the land and in the fields and not have direct contact with them.

We started to collect dolls and knitted outfits for them, as well as stuffed animals that were washable. A room in my house was set aside—it would come to be called the AIDS baby room—and it soon filled up with all sorts of washable toys and baby outfits, diapers, bottles, and even music boxes from Switzerland. It was almost like Christmas!

Anonymous letters began to arrive from mothers who were too afraid to let their community know they had AIDS and that their babies were dying of the dreaded disease. They simply wanted to tell another human being who was not afraid of their plight. We were unable to contact some of them because of the growing paranoia, much enforced by the churches, who not only expelled many AIDS patients but found it to be their "duty" to put blame and guilt on them. Little did they realize at that time that many young children became contaminated by blood transfusions they received early in life in order to keep them alive! Every AIDS patient was put in "the same basket": It was God's punishment for an immoral life-style and they deserved their suffering! A result of this hostility was the many letters that we received without our address and sometimes only signed with initials.

While we busily prepared for all the conceivable needs of these children, we applied for a rezoning of the five acres of my farmland where we planned to build the hospice. Then I was off to Europe to give a series of my five-day workshops and lectures, unsuspecting of the storm that was brewing in Virginia.

I was totally unaware that a man who had earlier worked on the construction of my log house, and had been fired by my construction foreman, had taken this opportunity for "sweet revenge." He went up and down the county collecting signatures on a petition to forbid the building of the hospice for AIDS babies. According to some people we interviewed later on, he presented it as a means of "importing AIDS" into the county. He even threatened another former construction worker who refused to sign the petition by "promising" the man he would never find a job in the county if he didn't sign. The Board of Supervisors apparently never questioned how or why two thousand out of twenty-eight hundred county residents signed such a petition within such a short time.

A public meeting was planned by my staff for October 9, 1985, and I returned from Europe to lend support and to answer whatever questions the people of Highland County, Virginia, might have. We left the farm in good spirits and were still very excited about the prospect of building such a haven for sick children. A last look at my animals—the burros, cattle, sheep, turkeys, chickens, ducks, and, last but not least, my adorable St. Bernard dog—convinced me that this was, indeed, the right place to house these babies.

When we reached Monterey, the county seat, the church was crowded with people, some of whom had arrived as much as an hour before the meeting was to start. It was only then that I was informed that the school board had notified us the day before that we would not be able to use the local school, which previously always held such meetings. No reason was given. I give credit to Paul McNutt, my office manager at that time, for going to the minister of the local Methodist church, who had the courage to say yes when we asked to use his church. Apparently no one else wanted us, but he was willing to stick his neck out and risk the ire of the community. I am sure that it will only be after his death that he will realize how much of that courageous choice will be credited in his "bookkeeping."

TV cameras were everywhere and reporters scrambled around with microphones trying to get seats near the podium where some of the experts were assembled. Rather than just telling the people about my own medical experiences with children with AIDS and the precautions in regard to this contagious disease, we invited six experts to answer questions from the audience:

Public Meeting: Monterey, Virginia
October 9, 1985

DR. KÜBLER-ROSS: There are many children dying of AIDS who have no toys, no love, no sunshine, no hugs, no

61

kisses, no loving environment. They are literally doomed to spend the rest of their lives until they die in those very expensive hospitals. And those are the children we would like to take care of. Before I move on, I need to tell you that those children are usually six months to two-and-a-half-year-olds. They will not be in touch with you. They do not go shopping. They don't use your schools. They stay on our place. We will have physicians and nurses and volunteers to take care of them. We have received many offers from literally all over the country, of physicians and nurses who would love to take care of these un-wanted, rejected, sick, terminally ill children. We also have a runway in front of the office for medical emergencies so we can fly them to the University of Virginia. We have our own food. We can obtain our own wood. We are self-supporting. We do not plan to cost the county much money. In fact, you will proba-bly get a lot of money from all the activities that will happen there. There are a lot of people who are worried about declining real estate values, about de-clining tourism, and that is as much of the fear as the first people had twenty years ago when we started the first hospice in the United States. What I am experiencing now with the fear from the resistance and the anxiety about helping dying children with AIDS is very familiar to me because I experienced that twenty years ago when I started working with dying patients. I was called a vulture. They spat in my face. I got a lot of hostility, some from doctors at the same institution. It is very familiar when people do something new that is not known, there is a lot of resistance, and a lot of fear. Once people know there is no danger to them—just like the hospices that are coming up now, almost like Chicken Delights all over the United States. It took us three years to start the first hospice twenty years ago. Now, every town has a hospice, and I don't think that any of you are afraid of these hospices. You are probably quite grateful that there are places to take care of your next of kin if you can't take care of them. So I will let Dr. Caplen* now share [with you] something about AIDS, and then we will [take] questions from you.

DR. CAPLEN: I'll try to make it brief because this room is probably going to get pretty hot with all these people in it. I have designed a brief statement here, which is divided into four main parts, and what I did was write in a few questions under each part with some answers. The four main parts will give you some general idea what the disease is about, I hope. The first thing I have here is the description of AIDS. *What is* AIDS? The name is an acronym which, probably most of you know by now, stands for "Acquired Immune Deficiency Syndrome." The definition of the disease—really it's any disease, which at least moderately—is a defect of some decreased immunity occurring in a person with no known cause of diminished resistance to that disease. That's kind of a textbook definition. More simply, as the name itself implies, it's the suppression of the body's normal ability to fight disease. *What is the cause of* AIDS? The cause of the virus is called HTLV-3, which is human T-cell

*Clifford Caplen, Staunton Health Department, Director, Central Shenandoah Health District.

lymphotrophic virus-3. And to define manifestation of this virus is [to say] that it is cytotoxic, or it kills what is known as the T-helper cells. The T-helper cells are important in our immune systems and this is what accounts for the breakdown of the patient's immune system and why we, in turn, cannot fight off diseases which normally we wouldn't be bothered with too much. *What are the symptoms of* AIDS? They have a variety of symptoms that have been loosely grouped under the heading of "AIDS-Related Complex" or ARC. I'm sure you have all heard of that. These include inexplicable persistence of fatigue, inexplicable fever, chills, or night sweats usually lasting for several weeks; inexplicable weight loss usually greater than ten pounds; swollen extrainguinal lymph nodes. These lymph nodes are usually in the neck or in the armpits. They are inexplicable in that they don't have any obvious cause. They generally last for more than two weeks. You will also see pink to purple flat or raised blotches which may occur under the skin, inside the mouth, nose, eyelids; initially they may resemble small bruises, but unlike bruises they do not disappear and the appearance of these, in at least a million Americans less than sixty years of age, is a rather ominous sign that this would go along with the actual case of AIDS. These people frequently have white spots, thrush, or candidiasis in their mouths, esophagus; blemishes in their mouths, little plaques called leukoplakia—more recently a little different than normal, called perileukoplakia. They have chronic diarrhea, a cough which has lasted too long to be attributed to a common respiratory infection, especially if it's accompanied by shortness of breath. It should be remembered that the presence of some or all of these symptoms does not necessarily imply that one has, or will develop, AIDS. And with the exception of those signs to indicate the presence of Kaposi's sarcoma, which is the presence of the bluish blotches I mentioned in a native-born American under sixty years of age, or of pneumonia secondary to pneumocystic carinii, which I mentioned is the shortness of breath, and that type of thing. These symptoms—other symptoms in that classification are simply a grouping of symptoms to help a physician bear in mind the possibility of AIDS existing in the particular patient he happens to have in front of him. These patients are also prone, because of their poor immune systems, to a variety of opportunistic infections. An opportunistic infection is a great many different types of infections which tend to occur much more frequently in people whose immune systems are disturbed because of AIDS or because of any other reasons. They may be under different types of treatment which temporarily depress their immune systems. Many of these are fungus-type organisms, atypical bacteria, herpes simplex, other things of that nature. The symptoms the patient shows at that time will not necessarily be the ones described under ARC but will generally be the symptoms of the particular opportunistic infection of the patient's experience. The most commonly associated diseases are pneumonia secondary to pneumocystic carinii and Kaposi's sarcoma, which accounts for approximately 57 percent and 19 percent, respectively, of all the opportunistic infections seen with AIDS. *How is* AIDS *transmitted?* It is generally stated that it is through intimate exposure to blood, blood-clotting secretions, and tissues of persons who have AIDS. The AIDS virus has been isolated from blood, semen, saliva, and tears, but there is no evidence so far of a case of AIDS having been transmitted by saliva or tears. From a practical point of view for the individual, AIDS is spread by sexual contact, IV drug use where needles are shared and are not sterile, to the newborn from an infected mother, and now rarely through blood transfusions as well as blood pack used in the treatment of hemophilia. This has become much more rare and will probably continue to become more rare due to the use of such things as heat-treated blood pack for hemophiliacs and the increased screening, including the AIDS virus-antibody testing, of the nation's blood supplies. *How is* AIDS *not transmitted?* There is no evidence at present that AIDS can be contracted through casual nonsexual contact with a person who has AIDS. Specifically, there is no evidence that AIDS is spread by an AIDS patient sneezing, coughing, or spitting; shaking hands or other nonsexual physical contact with an AIDS patient; contact with toilet seats, bathtubs, showers used by an infected person; contact with utensils, dishes, linens used by an infected person; eating food prepared or served by an infected person; contact with articles handled or worn by an infected person; and just being around an infected person even on a daily basis over a long period of time. *The treatment of* AIDS. There really is no treatment of the underlying condition. Treatment is directed toward whatever particular infection these individuals tend to come down with. The chance is

the neurological complications, the opportunistic infections that they tend to get. There are about a
dozen drugs that show some laboratory ability to control the AIDS virus. Testing humans thus far shows no
imminent breakthrough in treatment. All of the
drugs tried on human subjects so far have shown
toxicity problems to varying degrees, as well as varying degrees of effectiveness. The recent successful
inoculation of the disease in laboratory animals is
probably a helpful step forward in research on this
disease and, particularly, as I just mentioned, in experimental drugs. It gives you controlled conditions
under which you can treat animals and try to find out
the natural life cycle of this disease. One of the problems with the disease is that we are not really sure
what the natural life cycle of the disease is—what
happens to people with it. It's been around in Africa
for a number of years evidently—I don't know how
long—and I presume that we will eventually get
more information on this from that area of the world.
The last thing I mention is *prevention and public
education,* and this is the only method immediately
available to combat the spread of the disease. Since
sexual contact is a prime method of transmission, one
should know one's sexual contact well, limit one's
sexual contacts. Males should be sure to use condoms.
The diaphragm is probably of little use. Some of the
vaginal foams and jellies have not really been studied. Some people have said they may be of use, but
they will probably be of very limited value. Another
method of transmission is through exposure to blood
or body secretions of an infected person, so you
shouldn't share toothbrushes, or razors, with an in-

fected person. If there are blood-contaminated surfaces, the use of common household bleach, 5¼ percent sodium hyperchloride, diluted one to ten in water, is certainly sufficient to clean any particular surface. Wearing gloves is a commonsense approach to take, certainly if you have cuts on your hands, abrasions, that type of thing. As far as schools and day-care facilities are concerned, they should observe good hygiene for handling excrements and other body fluids. The virus has never really been isolated from any excrement—from urine, feces, that kind of thing. Attempts have been made; who knows, they may eventually isolate it. The virus is found in lymphocytes. Lymphocytes are frequently found in a lot of things—a lot of body fluids—so they may eventually find some small amounts in these discharges. They probably will never amount to anything to worry about in the way of infection because the virus itself is very labile: It doesn't stand up well when it is outside its own environment, which is inside our bodies. Similar in that respect to another lethal organism that we are much more familiar with, and that's rabies. Rabies is very deadly when it is in the body, too, but exposed to the outside world, it dries out and dies quite quickly. It appears that the AIDS virus is, likewise, rather fragile. As I was saying, good hygiene in schools and day-care facilities, and if the caretaker has cuts or abrasions on his hands, it probably makes common sense to wear gloves. The hand washing between and after caring for the children or cleaning soiled surfaces should probably be routine. Other helpful items are the use of disposable towels, use of disposable tissues. IV drug users should use clean, sterile needles; not share needles. In summary, I think we should not confuse the seriousness of this disease with the contagiousness. The average monogamous non-drug-using person would seem to have virtually no chance of becoming infected with AIDS. If there are any questions, that I can answer, I'll try to. I certainly don't know all of the answers. I may have to say, "I don't know."

Q: I would like to know if AIDS is out in the public in other countries?

DR. CAPLEN: Oh, yes, AIDS is pretty much a worldwide phenomenon. It's all through the European countries. As I said, it has been in certain African countries for many years now. It's not just the U.S.

Q: Did it start in their homosexual community, their heterosexual community, or how did it start?

DR. CAPLEN: With my limited knowledge on the history of this disease, it's my understanding it originally started in Africa. It originally came to people from monkeys. How that happened, I don't know. I'm not going to speculate on habits of certain people. I suspect that the virus underwent a certain type of mutant change or something of this nature and got into the human population. Unfortunately, with the generally poor health conditions in many of those countries, it has probably gone on for years not particularly recognized as being the disease that it is. One interesting thing is that the ratio of males to females in these areas is generally very close, basically females have it about as much as males do. In this country, at the present time, it is enormously much more common in males, but that's because, probably, it was mainly introduced into this country through the gay population.

Q: You say AIDS is not contagious? Why, in the hospitals, do they quarantine the patients or put them in isolation?

DR. CAPLEN: You have to remember we have two things here: we have the health-care worker, and we have the patient. The patient has an immune system that makes him less able to fight disease. He's more susceptible to all kinds of infections. Very frequently, when you see a nurse or some other health-care worker putting on a gown, cap, mask, that type of thing, it's to protect the patient, not to protect themselves. I might mention in this regard that they have done a study on about seventeen hundred health-care workers since 1983. Of that number in that period of time, they found twenty-six with positive serologies. All but three of them can be accounted for because of the life-style that those particular people lived. They were in high-risk groups. Of the three, one I don't know anything about, it's a confidential case of some kind; the other two basically got needle sticks and were infected through the blood.

Q: Dr. Caplen, I understand that there is a large corporation that requires its food handlers to have blood tests for AIDS now. And so does the U.S. Army. I wonder why they do that since it is not contagious.

DR. CAPLEN: You understand that I don't say AIDS is not contagious. AIDS is contagious, but mainly through certain ways. It is not thought to be contagious in any casual-type manner. Food handlers are not considered to be in a position to be passing along AIDS. I would probably assume that these people are under public pressure because of circumstances that arise when a condition like AIDS goes through the country and gets a lot of media attention. These people are a corporation. They're looking for a good public image. They surely don't want to have any problems develop. They're probably playing it as safe as they can. I would assume, on the basis of what I've said, they are being overcautious. I don't know that the U.S. Army is doing it.

Q: I read that on October 1 [*previous week*], the Defense Department has started requiring all recruits, army, navy, and marines, to take a blood test. Now, I'm sure they are relying on their reliable sources, Walter Reed Army Hospital, U.S. Naval Hospital, etcetera, before they started that. If this were not contagious, they wouldn't have to do that, and it would save the public a lot of money.

Q: Doctor, what will happen to these children in our country if nobody steps forward to care for them? And how are children like this cared for in countries where they have more experience with the disease?

DR. CAPLEN: In a whole variety of ways. I wouldn't say there is one uniform way for taking care of them. Dr. Ross will probably give you a better answer to that question as to where these children are being cared for now. They are probably in hospitals; they probably move on over to the welfare system, and are then placed, more than likely, in certain foster-

71

care settings. It's the way I would suspect it's been going on. She may be able to answer that better than me.

Q: I'd like to know why the doctor picked Highland County for this?

DR. CAPLEN: Would it be okay if I let her answer that?

Q: I'd like somebody to answer it!

DR. CAPLEN: Are there any other medical questions?

Q: As you speak I notice you say "has not been proven," "evidently"; there appears to be some sort of question. Could you answer specifically for us whether it's a fact or, in fact, it is suspicioned.

DR. CAPLEN: Well, it's the kind of fact you get from doctors and scientists. When you want absolutes, you are in the right place for it. You can get absolutes here [*indicating church*] but you can't get them from us because all we can give you is based on the best evidence that we have. I cannot guarantee any of these things to you.

Q: In other words, then, what you are saying is what you think—

DR. CAPLEN: Except it is not just what I think. It is what a lot of scientific studying has arrived at. See, actually, when you talk that way, we all live in uncertainty in every aspect of our lives. I don't know how to phrase this exactly, but nothing is for certain in this world. You know, grandfather goes to the post office over here, and somebody comes by for him and you say, "Well, he will be back in ten minutes." He may not. He may get hit by a car. He may have a heart attack. In that sense, nothing is for certain, so I'm not going to stand here and tell you absolutely 100 percent that you are not going to be able to transmit AIDS through tears. There is no evidence that this has occurred to date. It is an unlikely means of transmission. It, probably, is not going to occur, but I certainly couldn't guarantee it.

Q: But there is no evidence to the contrary either?

DR. CAPLEN: I don't think anybody has taken tears and tried to inoculate animals and reproduce the disease. It wouldn't be a fair test anyway, because you wouldn't normally be getting tears inoculated into your system or something like that. By the way, and I may not be completely accurate, I think that out of five or six patients, they found some tears in one, and I think, of another one or two, some possibility of the virus. These were very small inocula. You know, this disease doesn't have a high degree of transmissibility. It is not as high, for instance, as a sexually transmitted disease. You're more likely to catch gonorrhea from someone through intercourse than you are to catch AIDS. It doesn't have a high degree—

Q: I'm not interested in that—

DR. CAPLEN: Well, you might say that, but what I'm trying to get at is, it is not a highly contagious disease.

MR. N: I don't want those technical terms. I want the doctor to tell me why she picked Highland County for this thing!

DR. CAPLEN: She will.

DR. KÜBLER-ROSS Because I live in Highland County.

MR. N: Well, I want to tell you one thing. I heard on your program this morning through the news media that Highland County residents was ignorant of this disease. Which we are to a certain extent. We know as much about it as you do. You can't prove a thing. You haven't proven a thing.

DR. KÜBLER-ROSS What is your question?

MR. N: What is my question? Why are you coming to Highland County with this? Why are you disturbing all of these people, importing a disease in here that you know nothing about?

DR. KÜBLER-ROSS I am not importing a disease.

MR. N: Where in the hell are they coming from then? They ain't coming out of Highland County.

DR. KÜBLER-ROSS There are people in Virginia who have AIDS.

MR. N: They ain't in Highland County.

DR. KÜBLER-ROSS Wait a second—

REVEREND*: [*Interrupts loud and disorderly talk from audience*] Let us remember one thing: This is the House of God.

MR. N: Yes, sir. Yes, sir. I hope that I don't have to say nothing here. This is the wrong place to have this type of meeting anyway. I come to this county the

---

*Joseph H. Klotz, Jr., Minister, Monterey United Methodist Church.

same as you did. You been here, how long? Two years?

DR. KÜBLER-ROSS Yes.

MR. N: Two years. I came about the same time. You come here for a hospice thing. Why has this AIDS center entered into it now? I'm not saying a hospice is not a good thing, don't get me wrong.

DR. KÜBLER-ROSS We are here to help our fellow man— and needy children.

MR. N: You bringing in the children. What takes place is they go to the hospital where nobody don't care any- thing about them. Then they go to the Welfare, then to somebody like you. Highland County taxes will pay for that.

DR. KÜBLER-ROSS Highland County will not pay a penny.

MR. N: Aw, come on, you're talking about it will bring money into this county. I don't know where you get your figures at.

DR. KÜBLER-ROSS I have worked in this field with dying children for twenty years—

MR. N: People are dying every day.

DR. KÜBLER-ROSS Yes, but we help them.

MR. N: Help 'em die?

DR. KÜBLER-ROSS We help them live until they die.

Q: We have a good county here now. If this tragedy comes to our county, Dr. Ross, would you feel the least bit ashamed that you brought it to our county?

DR. KÜBLER-ROSS I think Jesus took care of leprosy patients two thousand years ago, and it's very, very important—

Q: Do you think you are Jesus?

DR. KÜBLER-ROSS No, I am not Jesus, but I am trying to do what was taught for two thousand years, and that is to love your fellow man, and help them.

Q: Won't you be ashamed—

DR. KÜBLER-ROSS I will not be ashamed of helping needy children.

Q: Dr. Ross, how would you compare leprosy with AIDS?

DR. KÜBLER-ROSS Leprosy is much more contagious than AIDS.

Q: Is that a fact? A proven fact?

DR. KÜBLER-ROSS Yes. Absolute fact.

Q: Dr. Ross, there are 4,651 cases of AIDS in New York alone; 131 cases in Virginia. This was from the September 23, 1985, edition of *Newsweek.* The question I have is actually a two-part question: Why not have it in New York where there is a great number of cases? Why put it in an isolated rural area and not put it closer to the people you serve? Why use a helicopter to transport them from Monterey to Charlottesville when you can locate in the heart of New York City and you can be closer to much more sophisticated, much more elaborate medical facilities. Many of these people die, such as Rock Hudson; now wouldn't it be better to have excellent medical facilities at hand, right immediately, rather than delay the period of time?

DR. KÜBLER-ROSS There will be places for these children all over the United States. Just like the first hospice was in one state and now there are hundreds all over the country. The more children there will be who are dying, or who don't get help, the more of these centers will pop up.

Q: Why do you not place the center in a place where it will be of the most value immediately? Why put them in this area?

DR. KÜBLER-ROSS Because I live here, and this is where I work.

Q: Why didn't you stay where you was at?

MR. N: I got a question for you. You coming into Highland County. There's no official in Highland County that knows you're coming. You've had the news media now for a month or better, from Washington, Roanoke, Richmond. They all know about it. We all know about it, but I haven't seen an official in Highland County step up here for or against this thing. I want to know why you haven't even applied for a permit. They don't even know you're coming in here. How is that ahappenin'?

DR. KÜBLER-ROSS We have filed a Notice of Intent with the Virginia Health Department. We are scheduled for filing for a rezoning permit which will begin about the seventeenth of this month, which would mean we will file our application with the Planning Commission.

MR. N: You haven't filed it yet though?

DR. KÜBLER-ROSS Not in this county yet.

MR. N: I understand that. Yeah. Okay. But since it hasn't been filed, these people that went out here and signed a petition to let you know that we do not need it in Highland County, and yet you're going to file for something like this to come in here and use the citizens of this county as guinea pigs. Is that your idea?

DR. KÜBLER-ROSS No.

MR. N: Well, it seems to be. I retired to come to this county to live out my life. I thought I was getting out of all this business when I come out of the city, but I think it's following me. I hate to see it but you're going to turn this place into a ghost town.

DR. MEYER*: I hear what you're saying and I'm not saying that everybody has to agree, but let me tell you about one case, and you're talking about you don't want it here—and if that stands, it stands. Then it will go some place else because these children have to be helped. Elisabeth lives here. And as far as I'm concerned, when children are dying and have no place to live and you're saying, "Don't let them touch me," then we have to look to see what's happening. Do you know that every single person in this room now is safe from getting AIDS through transfusion because one woman by the name of Helen Kushner, whose baby son died when he was transfused, refused to have the government shut her up and refused to

---

* Sandy Meyer, Ph.D., Human Behavior, one of Dr. Kübler-Ross's expert witnesses.

have the American Red Cross shut her up, and a long time ago HTLV-3 tests were available and when Helen's premature son, Sam, who was transfused in a hospital, got it; his twin sister, Sarah, did not. Three years later, Sam died, and Helen would not be quiet. Everybody told her to just be still, to sit down and shut up, and she went to the government and they said she was a hysterical mother, and she went to the Red Cross and they said, "Not our blood." Furthermore, they said, "We are not spending the five dollars to test it." This lady had the courage to face hostile crowds and hostile situations. I'm not trying to lump this crowd into one big thing, I understand there are strong passions—but I'm saying if we spend all night pointing fingers instead of trying to set up some kind of dialogue and to treat each other with dignity in that dialogue no matter how much we disagree, then I think we have reduced ourselves to a pathetic level. Helen Kushner had the courage to stand up. It's not that Highland County is the only place where this first home for AIDS babies can happen, but at least let us exchange information. You, with your concerns, and Dr. Kübler-Ross and Dr. Caplen and everybody else who are medical professionals . . . allow them to exchange their information with you, and see if there is any change. If there's no change, then there's no change. I don't think anybody's here to try to force-feed something down your throats.

[*Interruption from audience*]

DR. MEYER: Would you let me finish, please! Thank you. We are saying the children are abandoned. Children who are one year old, eighteen months old, have no place, not only to die; they have no place to live. This is a national tragedy, a national problem, and Highland County, and the county which I come from in Virginia, we are all part of this nation, so how, we, as a nation, choose to resolve the problem is fine, but to pretend it's not there, and to say, "Don't touch me with the national problem," it doesn't work that way, I'm sorry. In the county just south of here we have a case of a child with AIDS, and there are many more, so whether or not it's going to come to "your county" or not, it's already passed through. The children will be taken care of one way or another. But for the rest of this evening, we must remember we are in the House of God, in a House of Worship, and we must treat each [other] with dignity. I know that you have questions, but there are many people who have them also. We need to give them all a fair share.

Q: We have many a question, and if we have to set here all night, we are going to find out—

DR. MEYER: Please give your fellow community members a chance to speak—

Q: There are many concerns about AIDS, and there's a little concern about some of the facts that have been given here tonight concerning AIDS. I, for one, have been listening to programs on PBS; not much of a way to gain an education on the subject, but it's been shown that there aren't any scientific journals that are backing what you people are telling us about the contamination of AIDS. We know we have the least populated county east of the Mississippi. For that reason, we feel we are guinea pigs. Would you respond to that please.

80

DR. MEYER: I will again bring in Dr. Caplen with statistics, but I will say we have never had any case of intrafamilial spread, that means parents, kids, although it goes across the board. The parents and the siblings with children who have been afflicted with AIDS— none of the siblings nor the parents show positive in any of the AIDS tests. In the Kushner family, Sam, as children will, bit Sarah, his twin sister, and his father once. The tests show that the family had never been exposed to AIDS—parents eat after children, you know how that is. We taste the food and we trade back and forth. There is no sign of AIDS. The pediatrician who took care of Sam was four and a half months pregnant when she took over the case. She had absolutely no fear of touching Sam or that she could get it and pass it on to her child. She has been tested. Her son has been tested. They are both totally healthy. That is not from a scientific journal. I can only tell you that from the hands-on work that I've had the opportunity to do, every time we interact with any family, with any situation, we find that there is no intrafamilial spread. And there is more than shaking hands that is going on within a family.

Q: The question here though pertains to any ongoing studies: Why isn't this being done in a research facility as opposed to Highland County. I realize that this is just one more point on the graph that says there is no spread within the family—hopefully, in your group, there has been no spread. But still there is one more point; there has not been a conclusion drawn that has been published. You can state facts based upon your experience, but we are worried about whether the facts are based upon the entire scientific community's experience; we don't just want single points from your experience, and those haven't been published. Furthermore, there isn't much going on with that type of research that we are aware of. Now, if you're aware of it, we would like to know.

DR. MEYER: This is Dr. Babb,* whose son died from AIDS—

DR. BABB: To relieve some of your fears, I'd have to say that I'm sorta from this area. My family comes from Petersburg, West Virginia, right up the road here, about fifty miles, and I grew up and got my education while I was living over in West Virginia. I graduated from the Medical College of Virginia, in Richmond, in 1941. I used to drive through here, on Route 250, so I am not such a stranger. We are not all from New York. I want to congratulate the community—I had no idea there were so many people in Monterey— and certainly you are not indifferent. You are to be congratulated on your interest shown in this meeting. From this discussion, I would first like to say two things: one, you say that Monterey, if we have this facility, will suffer in its reputation, and become a ghost town. I can tell you that Monterey will suffer a great deal more in its reputation if you reject this request.

[*Adverse verbal reaction from the audience*]

DR. BABB: This is just my opinion. I would like to reply to another remark from someone in the back of the

*Donald F. Babb, Pathologist (retired), expert witness for Kübler-Ross.

audience. In regard to the army testing recruits for the AIDS antibodies, I've had a lot of experience as an army physician during the war, admitting recruits from the National Guard, etcetera, and they always did tests for syphilis and other tests, and why did they do that? Because once the recruit is in the army, the army is responsible for his medical care the rest of his life, and their fear is possibly not that the soldier will transmit the disease to his fellow soldiers, but that the United States Government will, then, be responsible for his disease, if he comes down with AIDS in the army. I think that's the reason that the army is required to test recruits—not the danger of contagion. And our friend here that says there is not any scientific evidence published about it, there is a recent review of the epidemiology in the *Journal of Science* which, for October, I don't have the exact date, I am sure you can find it in any well-furnished library; that's a reputable journal. There's a review in there by a committee that represents all of the scientific organizations in the United States and their conclusions are exactly the same as you have been told here by Dr. Caplen, that there is no casual transmission of AIDS, and all other medical doctrines come from experience. We have no other way to form medical opinions and all we can ever say in any disease, is "in our experience this doesn't happen," and this disease is being studied intensively by great scientific institutions. My own contact has been principally with the National Institute of Health. They, I am sure, know more about it than anybody else, and I talked to Dr. Clifford Lane this morning, who is in charge of a great many of the AIDS programs they have. They have continuous programs in which they are using drugs on an experimental basis on large numbers of AIDS patients, and there they discovered and demonstrated the virus that causes AIDS. They identified it. They have the virus. Now, they have been able to inject the virus into primates so that they can— I don't think that there is any doubt that within a few years, there will be a cure for AIDS. But the conclusion of all the scientific evidence has been that AIDS is not transmitted by any casual contact and that, basically, the only transmission is where you have something that is similar to blood or one of the body fluids extracted from the patient who has the disease and it is injected in some way, in contact with the circulation of the patient who is infected.

Q: On the question of tissue exchange and blood exchange, does that include insect to man?

DR. BABB: There is absolutely no evidence that this is an insect-borne disease. Now, remember, one criterion that medical science uses in determining the cause of the disease is the epidemiology of the disease. What is the pattern of its spread? If there were a pattern of spread of disease by insects such as there is, for example, in Africa, where we have the young African children with massive swelling tumors, mainly in the jaw, it is a somewhat similar disease. It is caused by a virus, no insect factor has ever been identified or proved, but the epidemiology, the location in which the disease occurs in lower lying, very warm areas where there are mosquito-borne diseases, that's from the epidemiology, the way it is spread, and the way it is located. Now, if this were so in AIDS, we would see a different pattern of the grouping of the cases, so there is no evidence that it is transmitted by insects.

Q: Do you think a child who has AIDS can be cared for properly until he dies the way that Dr. Ross plans to care for him?

DR. BABB: Oh, definitely, I certainly do. Let me just give you my experience. That's the reason they brought me here.

Q: I'm still asking about why the army is testing recruits for AIDS if it's not contagious.

DR. BABB: It's a logical conclusion that the army has to know—the first thing that a recruit gets is a complete physical examination because the army doesn't want to admit anybody that has any diseases. They take an X ray for tuberculosis. They take numerous samples of blood, and the idea of that is that you don't have a service-related disability later that you had when you came into the army. That's the only reason that I can see for it. I'm not familiar with the army's processing—I don't know if they make this test when the recruit first appears before he signs the papers. I don't know those details.

Q: Since there is not a cure for AIDS, it also means that it will spread as well, doesn't it?

DR. BABB: You're assuming that. I think that my explanation is a little more logical. You all are too young to remember, but when we used to have tuberculosis— I'm sure you had people with tuberculosis here—it was much more infectious than AIDS. There's no

85

comparison and you isolated them, but there was not this unreasonable fear of that disease that we have in this case. The incubation period is— I do not know, and it is not possible that anybody can have enough statistics to tell you what is the average time for a serological test to change from negative to positive. I don't think that we have experience in enough cases in which we can say the exact time of the inoculation because if you didn't do a test, you didn't know. You can't hide from AIDS. It will come to Highland County, but it will not come from these children. What are you going to do, put a border up here and examine everybody that comes in? It's impossible. With the rate that AIDS is occurring, sooner or later someone from this county will have it. It won't be from these children. It will be from adult sexual contacts.

Q: Dr. Ross, I'd like to ask you a question about your sewage system. How come your sewage system is so inadequate now that you truck it down to Monterey and dump it in the creek? If you are so concerned about human beings and disease and all of that—

PAUL: [Dr. Kübler-Ross's temporary office manager] I'd like to respond to that, if I may. We are not trucking, nor have we attempted to truck, any sewage to Monterey or anywhere else. We have been approved by the Virginia State Water Control Board for a sewer system. It is not put in because presently what we have is on septic systems.

Q: If Dr. Ross is so interested in cancer, how come she sprays herbicides on the field before she plants alfalfa? You know herbicides have been proven to cause cancer.

PAUL: Can we take one at a time? As far as putting herbicides on the field, this is done, of course, with the recommendation of the Soil Conservation Service—

Q: If she cared so much about people with cancer, and people with AIDS, she wouldn't spray herbicides on her field to plant alfalfa. She doesn't care. Something is not coming down right in this county. It's supposed to be a government of the people, by the people. These people don't want this thing and the government officials should realize that and not have it.

PAUL: I agree with you on that point because if they don't want it, we can't do anything in this county. We can't proceed any further than we are right now unless the County Board of Supervisors approves it.

Q: How about the people? We are the County Board of Supervisors.

PAUL: You are the County Board of Supervisors, that is correct. And you are speaking—and I'm sure they will hear it—but as you said we are a democracy—

Q: What about the herbicides?

PAUL: The Soil Conservation Service recommended it. I can't address that any other way.

Q: I want to know if you have filed your application with the state for a Certificate of Need.

PAUL: We have not applied.

Q: What have you applied for?

PAUL: We have only filed a notice of intent with the state.

Q: What is the next step?

PAUL: The next step is to file with the county for rezoning.

Q: You are required by the State Board of Health to receive a Certificate of Need to operate your AIDS center before you will be able to go into operation.

PAUL: We have a little bit of a conflict between the state and the county. We were advised by the county that we could not submit an application for rezoning until we were licensed by the state. Then we went to the state and they said, I believe rightly so, "We can't license you until you're properly zoned, until your plans are complete, until this has all been submitted and approved"—and that's where we are now.

Q: I've got a couple of questions. First off, I want to thank Dr. Ross for coming here. I want to know a little about your air transportation—how you're going to handle everything? Will you have facilities on hand? Or will you require the helicopter from Charlottesville to come over and pick the children up?

DR. KÜBLER-ROSS: I am only referring to the runway that we have in front of our office because we have been warned that if we ever needed ambulance service they will refuse to come and put those children in their ambulance. So I said if that's their choice, I will accept that. They are responsible for their own choices. We have our own cars, and we happen to have a runway in front of the office, and somebody has already volunteered with an airplane and a pilot, to bring those children, if necessary, to the University of Virginia, where I happen to have a professorship, where naturally we will get good treatment for those children. We will have our own oxygen and our own medical equipment. This is only for the real hot emergency if a child needs immediate hospitalization.

Q: I have one other question: If this is not approved by the Board of Supervisors, then you don't plan to come here? Not just put it "on the back burner." Some people have said they really don't care, but we have had quite a few calls saying that they do not want it in this county.

DR. KÜBLER-ROSS: But I tell you, and I really mean it, when we started our first hospice, we got the same phone calls, and then everybody wanted to buy land nearby because all the doctors needed housing, all the nurses needed housing, and just the opposite came true.

Q: Okay, but AIDS is not the same as cancer. What I am talking about is everybody is scared about it. I am talking about fear. How do you answer these people who firmly believe that tourists are not going to come to the county; that because of AIDS, the attendance at the Maple Festival may very well drop next year. The Chamber of Commerce, residents, everybody is talking.

DR. KÜBLER-ROSS: You see, I can't see it because I don't believe it.

Q: I'd like to ask Dr. Ross if she knows of anyone in this country who has offered to build such a place for these dying children.

DR. KÜBLER-ROSS: There are several offers that have come in during the past week and since I've just come back from Europe. I haven't read all the mail, but the nearest offer I've received came yesterday from Staunton [Virginia].

Q: What we want from you is a guarantee that you will not pollute our water system, our sewer system with AIDS. We want a guarantee from you that it will stay on your farm and that it will not go anywhere in the county other than that, and that it will not affect any tourism, any property values, anything like that. We don't want it because it will affect our lives, regardless of whether we catch it or not. It's going to come into the county; yes, we will eventually get it, but we don't want it imported in here. Let it come in on its own. That's what we want from you, that our whole world is not going to be disrupted because of your facility.

DR. KÜBLER-ROSS: I cannot give you any guarantee—

Q: Then we do not want it if you cannot give any guarantees.

DR. KÜBLER-ROSS: I am just telling you that—

Q: I would like to ask you, Can you deny that AIDS can destroy the human race? Can you deny that?

DR. KÜBLER-ROSS: If there is no more promiscuity, no more bisexual men, and no more IV drug-using people, this disease can be eradicated.

Q: You're saying that this started in Africa with the homosexuals and drug users—

DR. KÜBLER-ROSS: No, I'm talking about the Western world.

Q: You cannot deny that it is a dread disease?

DR. KÜBLER-ROSS: It is a dread disease.

Q: And it is the only disease which we know of that destroys the immune system?

DR. KÜBLER-ROSS: It is dreaded. It is not the only disease that affects the immune system, and even by the most pessimistic predictions, nobody has ever predicted that it is capable of destroying the human race.

Q: I still go back to the countries where it started. How did it get there? Was it by these methods? It must have gotten there some way. I still don't know how it got across the seas. It must have changed its form. What's to say it won't change its form again?

DR. MEYER: The most popular theory is that it came from monkeys in Africa. They are doing other research right now, including some problems with our blood bank. They have started doing investigative work trying to pinpoint exactly what happened and how it got transferred. One that most of you are aware of is from monkeys. It is not homosexually spread that way. It is spread because some of the tribes eat monkeys. That's really how they think it happened. We are also concerned that once it's spread over there, there is a problem with the blood bank and the way we use that. That is not scientifically proven. It is just something that they are right now doing investigative work on. Since this is a democracy, let's take a vote right now and see how the residents of Highland County feel about having this in our county.

Q: You say we are ignorant. There isn't a home in the county that doesn't have a TV or radio. . . . These people are well educated. Don't treat us like we are ignorant!

Q: I have heard all of the arguments that have been going on here tonight. We think it is contagious and you don't. We are not going to settle this issue tonight because we are at odds. You have said that you have had hospices for years, that you have children there to teach them to live until they die. Is that right?

DR. KÜBLER-ROSS: To help them live until they die.

Q: I would like to know how do you teach them to live until they die. Do you teach them to die in Jesus Christ? Or do you teach them reincarnation? Are you bringing a cult into this area?

DR. KÜBLER-ROSS: I am a Christian, and I am not bringing a cult into this area.

Q: Excuse me, I didn't hear that.

DR. KÜBLER-ROSS: I am a Christian and I am not bringing a cult into this area.

Q: Dr. Ross, in your future plans, do you have any plans to bring adults, homosexuals with AIDS, to your care center?

DR. KÜBLER-ROSS: We have no such plans.

Q: So far?

DR. KÜBLER-ROSS: Right.

Q: Why is it important that these children be cared for in the way you want to care for them as they die?

DR. KÜBLER-ROSS: If you had a child who was dying and you couldn't take care of him or her, wouldn't you want somebody to hold him, hug him, and love him?

Q: And this is why you want to bring the children here?

DR. KÜBLER-ROSS: Yes.

Q: Doctor, you said you had a personal experience with AIDS. I'd like to know what it's like when a child dies.

DR. BABB: My personal experience was not with an infant. My son died of AIDS about one year ago in the University Hospital in Charlottesville, and I'm glad to say that he was never rejected by his family because of abnormal fear of the disease. He lived with us, my wife and I and his brother, for about eighteen months after he was diagnosed with the disease. He was treated at all of the best medical centers with all of the medical treatments that were available, and as far as his being at home, we never treated him any differently than when he didn't have the disease. Of course, we used normal hygienic practices, which everybody should always use. We didn't use each other's toothbrushes or razors, we washed the dishes, and we washed our hands, but that's as far as it went. All of us have been tested for the possibility of this contagion, and there is no evidence—of course, as we understand it, the disease may have a very long incubation period. I can't guarantee that I won't have AIDS sometime, but I have no fear of it—the way my son was treated in the hospitals and the National Institute of Health and in the University Hospital at Charlottesville. They have experience with treating AIDS. He was in isolation while he was there. Part of this, as was explained by the doctor previously, was because the AIDS patient has to be protected from contamination with other people, but it is only logical when a hospital uses an isolation technique that is perfectly reasonable and logical, by the people, the nurses, the doctors—and my largest experience was with those in the National Institute of Health where I stayed; they know more about this disease than any place else. They do not have what I am sure is an unreasonable fear of the disease. They know how it is transmitted. They take the precautions that are necessary, but as far as the transmission of the disease from these children, I think that there is no reasonable possibility that it will occur.

Q: You see this as a possibility for Highland County to be a good samaritan?

DR. BABB: I certainly do. I think that your reputation will suffer a great deal more if you refuse it than if you take it.

Q: When they bring these children out here and if they cut themselves and our children come in contact with them, will our children have it, too?

DR. KÜBLER-ROSS: You have to know that these children are babies from six months to two and a half years old, and unless you choose to bring your children to my place and play with them, you will never ever, ever have any physical contact with them. We have

94

many brothers and sisters of siblings who have had AIDS who lived together in the same household for two years until they died. They had bloody noses and the usual scratches, and those children are still well now after three and a half years.

Q: I read somewhere that the incubation period is five years. How can you say that they won't get it.

DR. KÜBLER-ROSS: That is for grown-ups. Young children's time is much shorter because they get the disease through the womb.

Q: I'm asking the question about an open cut.

DR. KÜBLER-ROSS: Yes, but with little children, the incubation time is usually much briefer than with grown-ups.

Q: Dr. Ross, you're talking about taking children from six months to two and a half years. What kind of guarantee would you give us that you wouldn't bring older children, which you would then try to put into the home.

DR. KÜBLER-ROSS: The older children—that's a totally different group of children. The only older children that I know of, and there are lots of them, are hemophiliacs, and because of the hemophilia, they got lots of blood transfusions and they got the AIDS through them, and those are the children of intact families, so I would not consider taking older children for that reason.

Q: Dr. Ross, all of the support that you have seems to be coming from California, so why don't you take the AIDS children with you to California?

DR. KÜBLER-ROSS: If you have the time, come to my house and look—

Q: I don't want to come to your house!

DR. KÜBLER-ROSS: My support comes from all over the world.

Q: From the paper that we got hold of we got the impression that you're treating patients at your center already. In your news broadcast a few weeks back you said you'd be asking for one hundred dollars from the citizens of Highland County, but tonight you said that you wouldn't ask Highland County for any money. Why are you saying now that you don't want any money?

DR. KÜBLER-ROSS: If you want to donate, I would not say no.

Q: You came here two years ago, and now you think you can rule the county—

Q: We are concerned people to the point that we have you people standing here telling us one thing and the media telling us something else. Frankly, we don't quite believe you, so the question here is, when you first started applying for a hospice over here in Headwaters there was no mention about the AIDS program, I'd like to hear from the representative from the Department of Health again on the limitations of your license should it be applied for—whether the Highland County residents want it or not, we want to be sure we can't be skirted around.

DR. MEYER: Dr. Caplen is not here right now.

96

Q: If you can get the money, what's going to stop you from going on and taking grown-ups with AIDS?

DR. KÜBLER-ROSS: There are lots of people who take grown-ups who have AIDS.

Q: So why didn't you talk about AIDS babies when you came here?

DR. KÜBLER-ROSS: Two years ago, when I came here, we wanted to start a workshop and training center and include a facility for dying children.

Q: Why, when you were starting, did you not say you wanted a facility for AIDS children?

DR. KÜBLER-ROSS: In those days, there was no need for taking them—this is a totally new phenomenon. It is only in the last year and a half that the first children in the U.S. have been dumped in hospitals with the mothers leaving without having a forwarding address. It is only within the last few months that we became aware that this is a national problem.

DR. TAYLOR: (one of Dr. Ross's expert witnesses) I am Dr. Henry Taylor. I work in Franklin, West Virginia. I am an internist. I am the only internist physician on Dr. Ross's Board of Directors, so I'm here as a representative of the board. When Elisabeth first came here, she was talking, first, about a training site and a conference center. At that time, the issue about caring for children who were dying was raised. The issue of AIDS was first brought into— I don't know when Elisabeth started getting concerned about it, but it was brought up at the board meeting in June. I think it is important for people to realize that part of this discussion—and people are saying you haven't applied for an application, you haven't done this, you haven't done that; what are your plans, what are your details— The board has been concerned because there are a lot of people on the board who are from here. I'm living down the street, if not in Highland County, and Elisabeth is concerned about community reaction. As she says, she has been through this with the whole issue of hospices and death and dying. Part of why we're having this meeting and getting the discussion going is because there should be dynamic interaction. That is what I feel as a board member. I have not talked to Elisabeth about it so far, so the applications are not in. The discussions are good, I think, coming up now before it comes up to the Board of Supervisors. If we had sprung this meeting on you two days before the Board of Supervisors, I think that would have been very unfair. Elisabeth is doing this because there is a concern. My understanding—and I would like Elisabeth to comment on this, about what is the purpose of the Center for AIDS—my understanding is, based on my review of the literature, is that there are children who are orphaned, toddlers with AIDS. They are abandoned. We aren't talking about siblings or other family members, and part of the purpose of this is continuing in the spirit of education and training of other staff people—not necessarily to do all the care here. Currently there is very little work done to train people like myself, to train the doctors—I mean, we are calling in people from other places to give information about AIDS here. It's because medical personnel don't know a lot about it.

Q: A few years ago people tried to get a nursing home here, and the reason they said we couldn't have one was because we didn't have the medical facilities. If we don't have the medical facilities for something like that, how can we have them for AIDS? I mean, if you have terminally ill children, you have to rush them to the hospital. I would object to having them use our rescue squad.

DR. TAYLOR: I think that's one reason Elisabeth didn't answer the question about details, and I think that's a very valid question. Those details are continuing to be worked on. We are talking about a relatively limited number of people and developing a system and only handling the children which can be handled. That's different than a nursing home. I work at a nursing home in Pendleton County, which has a very different set of requirements.

Q: Her facilities will be built to take care of the children as they are taken in—

DR. TAYLOR: Yes, and that is the reason why the details cannot be given at this time. It will take a lot of work, but as a concerned board member, I can tell you we are hearing these concerns, and dialogue and discussion can go on, and planning can go on. It depends on what the requirements are. There are some places that say, "Sure, we will let the Rescue Squad do it." The Rescue Squad doesn't want to do it and I appreciate the limitations. In Pendleton County, I am aware of the resources and limitations, but I am part of those resources. I don't think the board or Elisabeth are going about it with that intent.

DR. KÜBLER-ROSS: We're going to have twenty-four-hour coverage with physicians.

Q: Dr. Ross, what educational facilities are you going to have?

DR. KÜBLER-ROSS: Six months to two-and-a-half-year-old children don't need any school education. They are preschool children and toddlers.

Q: I am the building and zoning administrator. And there's only one official that deals with this at the start and that's me. I work for the county and also represent these people, but I've got to remain neutral. I'm right on the fence line.
[*Much audience reaction! Applause!*]

MR. N: You're right in the middle, right? What side of the fence are you going to fall on?
[*More audience reaction! Applause!*]

Q: Okay, it's going to take you a year to a year and a half to build your facility. What's going to happen to the ones lying in the hospitals dying now?

DR. KÜBLER-ROSS: But by next year there will be twice as many.

Q: That's right, they'll double, so why bring them here? Why not keep it in New York, or wherever they're coming from? Where you have your facilities— Why do you have to fly them to Charlottesville when they can be driven down the street to the nearest hospital. It's an hour and a half to Staunton to King's Daughter's Hospital by ambulance. I know. I ride in it almost every other day.

100

DR. KÜBLER-ROSS: Just because our hospital facilities are there and I'm on the staff.

Q: I have a question for Dr. Taylor, how do the people in Pendleton County feel about this?

DR. TAYLOR: I know there has been a lot of concern here in Highland County. I have heard some talk, rumors, going around. I don't really think I'm a fair judge because I'm clearly identified as being on the board. I've heard things go both ways. In the county where I work, we have a series of classes and education. People are asking questions. People are asking not only because of what's happening here, but because of what they hear on TV and all the information that is being mentioned. We are planning to continue having classes. I'm keeping up. I know that people are concerned; they want to make sure that there are adequate safeguards.

Q: Dr. Babb, was your son cremated or buried?

DR. BABB: He was cremated.

Q: If people die of AIDS and are not cremated, how are the body fluids disposed of, and how will these children be disposed of?

DR. BABB: I am going to explain why my son was cremated. He was born and raised in Puerto Rico. I practiced medicine for forty years in Puerto Rico. That was his home and we wanted to take him back there and bury him, so that was the most simple way of doing it. It was not because of the need to do it. On the other hand, as a pathologist, which I am and I've had a lot of experience with dead bodies, in a normal

101

embalming procedure, the solution used will certainly kill all AIDS virus.

Q: Formalene doesn't kill foot disease in sheep.

DR. BABB: This is not foot rot in sheep!

Q: I love children, but the mothers that have abandoned these children are out using drugs, having sexual relations, and bringing forth more children?

DR. KÜBLER-ROSS: Probably.

DR. BABB: Certainly we ought to admit that some of our resentment against this disease is to try to punish people who have illicit sexual relations—I don't think that should be. That wasn't a question, that was a statement.

Q: Dr. Ross, I notice that you use the present tense: "I am not planning," "I am not interested." But that implies to me that, "I am not planning now, but I might plan in the future"; "I am not interested now, but I could be interested in the future." The possibilities that this could be a full-fledged facility for all homosexuals, regardless of their ages. This is a problem that I'm concerned about as a schoolteacher—contaminating the other students—but the main thing is, can you promise us that you will *never* have a program that ministers and serves people over the age of two and a half years?

DR. KÜBLER-ROSS: I cannot promise anything. I have to be very honest. If somebody would have told me twenty years ago that I would work with dying children, I would have said, "No way will I work with dying children." If they had asked me five years ago, "Are you going to have a center for AIDS babies," I would have said, "No way, how do I know anything about AIDS babies." I have always helped the neediest population. My main speciality is that of young children, and as I said to somebody here who asked about school children, all the AIDS children that I know who are of school age are hemophiliacs who are taken care of by their families. And no natural parents would leave their children in Highland County if they lived in Staunton or somewhere else because they do want the daily contact with them. I only want to help the rejected children who get the disease in the first months—not years—of their lives. Their life expectancy is such that the probability that any of our children will ever reach school age—until there is a cure found, naturally—is nil.

Q: I am a born-again Christian. I believe with all my heart that we ought to serve these children, but I believe that it ought to be in the area of New York or San Francisco first. Now, eventually, when we have the problem here, then we should bring them here. We ought to serve New York and San Francisco first. Let them develop a center there.

DR. KÜBLER-ROSS: Mother Teresa is now starting a center to help those patients in New York City.

Q: Then why don't you go to New York City?

Q: If you should decide with the majority of the people here not to have AIDS children here, would you go ahead and have a hospice for elderly people and other children with noncommunicable diseases?

103

DR. KÜBLER-ROSS: Would I proceed with such a hospice? If I find a place where those AIDS babies will be taken care of, I would be happy to, but we have to find a place to help those AIDS babies.

Q: I would like to know who is going to be responsible for seeing about the health of this center. Would it be under the Health Department, or under state supervision, or who would oversee it?

DR. KÜBLER-ROSS: Actually, it is the State Health Department that oversees it.

DR. TAYLOR: Licensing does come from the State Health Department so the State Health Department is responsible for enforcing regulations.

Q: I think Dr. Ross answered a lot of our questions and concerns when she said she couldn't promise anything.
[*Loud response from audience! Applause.*]

DR. MEYER: Should there be a change of heart—and I'm not saying there will be, I'm just saying should there be—all the money that will be solicited for this particular project would have to be spent completely on this specific project; that's the way that type of money is raised, and so that, in itself, would preclude that, in this area, it could expand beyond that. Questions from this lady and this gentleman, and they will be the final two for this evening.

Q: I just want to say, Thank God for Dr. Ross, whether people agree with her or not. People are frightened, we can understand that, but in order to become unfrightened, we must become enlightened. I had a

brother with tuberculosis who spent seven years in a
sanatorium. When I went to visit him, there were
bars on the windows. If that were now, that he was
having that disease, and there was a lady like Dr. Ross
taking care of him, there would be no bars, there
would be no isolation, there would be contact and
love, and that's what we need. Whether you agree
with the doctor or not, it's your opinion, but I say
thank you for giving us a chance to ask questions, and
I say, God bless you.
[*Big applause!*]

Q: You mentioned fears and threats, and I am wondering,
with the level of fear in the county, whether your
center or anybody has been receiving threats here,
saying, "Don't do this, or things will happen."

DR. KÜBLER-ROSS: I haven't received any threats. Not yet.

DR. MEYER: We thank the pastor of this church for letting
us assemble here, and you for your comments. Good
night.

The meeting was over late at night, and the local
people dispersed slowly and, most of them, angrily. They
were annoyed at the news coverage, which, many felt,
prevented them from expressing their real anger. They
were annoyed that it was held in a church, which prevented some of them from using the language they would
have liked to use. But there were also a few who just
silently shook their heads and whispered, "I'm sorry." A
group of people from an adjacent little community came
over and rather publicly expressed their support.

When we left in a small caravan of cars, a County Sheriff's car pulled up in front of us and one followed all over the mountain to our farm. We waved good-bye to them, but they ignored our signal of appreciation.

There was a period of passive resistance, unfriendliness, and a long exchange of letters written to the local newspapers. Little notes from supporters who did not dare speak up in the public meeting appeared in our mailbox. Drivers of trucks that usually passed us on the road with a friendly, neighborly wave of the hand, stopped waving. Suddenly we had become persona non grata in the community. A local member of my Board of Directors asked to be excused from serving on it.

Chapter 5

Letters to the Editor

September 9, 1985

Editor:

I am writing you to ask how many Highland County residents are in favor of the AIDS center being located in our county.

Why should we bring a disease such as this to our county? Many residents know little or nothing about this disease.

They say we can't locate a nursing home at the Jack Mountain Village area due to the distance of the nearby hospitals. Well, just what do they expect to do for a hospital for the children at the center if a real emergency should arise?

Our supervisors have performed a terrific job in getting a company to locate at the former Aileen plant and created jobs for area people, so why not bring something else to Highland to create more jobs instead of an AIDS center. How many people do you expect to work around such a contagious disease? I won't.

Highland has been a place for city people to retire and move to our county to get away from the hectic city life. I am a life long resident of Highland and hope to be able to stay here for my lifetime, but with bringing such disease as this to our county it just makes me want to move.

I hope our supervisors will do everything in their power to keep AIDS from coming to our county.

I strongly oppose the AIDS center.

A. L.
Monterey, Virginia

September 9, 1985

Editor:

The announcement of Dr. Elisabeth Kübler-Ross's plan to operate a center for AIDS children seems to be generating a great deal of heat, but very little light. Perhaps we should get some facts before the public.

Scientifically, AIDS can be spread only by transfer of bodily fluids from a patient to a well person. Thus far the only documented cases of transmission of AIDS have been through kissing, intimate sexual contact, and blood transfusions. Theoretically, a physician or nurse who accidentally injures himself with a needle used to inoculate an AIDS patient could get the disease, but this is not known to have happened. Dentists have also been advised to wear goggles, masks, and gloves when working in the mouths of AIDS patients, although there have been no cases of transmission to dentists.

What we are certain of is that there is no danger from simply being with these patients. In AIDS wards in various hospitals, there has never been a case of a physician, nurse, or ward aid contracting the disease by caring for the patients.

It is a very beautiful and compassionate thing that Dr. Elisabeth Kübler-Ross plans to do. I hope that the good people of Highland County will not oppose this through lack of knowledge of the facts.

F. C. S., M.D.
Monterey, Virginia

September 13, 1985

Editor:

I am writing in reply to the letter of F. C. S., M.D., of Monterey, concerning Dr. Elisabeth Kübler-Ross's plan to operate a center for AIDS children in Highland County.

Dr. S. stated there seems to be a great deal of heat, but very little light, and we should get the facts before the public. I will agree with that 100 percent, but we must face the fact there is little known about AIDS, and no cure, as of now, has been found.

As he stated in his letter, one way AIDS could be spread is by bodily fluids from the patient to the well person through kissing. Now, we all know that children will put things in their mouth and other children will pick the same object up and put it in their mouths. They eat after each other and play with toys that have the AIDS germs on them.

If it has been advised that dentists wear goggles and masks and gloves to work in the mouths of AIDS patients, then I don't think we need such a disease in Highland County.

We all know that the children will have to be treated for the disease, but I can't see bringing children from places like New York and other large cities to places like Highland County to be treated.

I also read the letter to the editor from A. L. of Monterey. I agree with her 100 percent, and I will never agree to an AIDS center being built in Highland County. I do not think it is the right place for such a center, and I hope our supervisors will take a hard look at the problem and oppose it.

There are very few places in the country that people can enjoy good country living and Highland County is one of them. Let's keep it that way. Let's oppose the AIDS center in Highland County.

E. F.

September 13, 1985

Editor:

Considering I obviously was one source of heat without light, I feel the need to respond to a letter written by Dr. F. C. S.

This letter is not intended to condemn, degrade, or criticize anyone. I do, however, wish to ask some questions and state my views concerning the proposed AIDS care center near Headwaters.

The statement declaring the complete impossibility of contracting AIDS by casual contact worries me. How can our doctor make such a statement? Upon whose authority or what material does he make that guarantee? I have yet to see an official document declaring that as truth. Has the disease control center in Atlanta made some discovery that I haven't seen or heard? Even Dr. Kübler-Ross admits there is no 100 percent guarantee.

Reading newspaper accounts, watching news clips, and talking with people in the medical field, one thing stands out—AIDS patients are immediately isolated from other patients. Their doctors and nurses wear gloves, gowns, and masks. Doesn't sound like a noncontagious disease as diabetes or kidney disease [, with patients] allowed to visit their neighbors or walk in halls. No gloves, masks, or fears! Why? Do those doctors and nurses know something we and our doctor don't?

At the risk of being considered cruel and heartless, I must stand opposed to the AIDS center. I cannot in good conscience support anything that would risk the health of the citizens or economic future of Highland County.

H. M.
McDowell, Virginia

September 16, 1985

Editor:

A disturbing polarization appears to be forming in the community over the center proposed by Dr. Elisabeth Kübler-Ross for the care of children with AIDS. It is hoped that opinions of support or opposition can be based on facts rather than emotional responses.

Dr. Kübler-Ross and Dr. F. C. S. both quite accurately quote the lay press citing the remote possibility of contracting the disease through casual contact. Those of us who have had the privileged responsibility of caring for small children know that there is no such thing as "casual contact," what with runny noses, projectile vomiting, copious tears, and dirty diapers. Recognized authorities in centers of AIDS research of the disease is quite superficial. Unfortunately, known facts seldom reassure the public when they perceive a threat to their health. One need only cite the case of leprosy, which has been shunned for centuries and is probably much less contagious than AIDS.

Dr. Kübler-Ross is a recognized authority on death and dying. We know nothing of her expertise in communicable diseases or pediatrics. As of this date she is the only visible health-care professional identified with her staff. The scarcity of medical and paramedical personnel in this area is well known. Dr. Kübler-Ross is quoted by the Staunton *News-Leader* as saying, "There will be physicians at the center." How often, from where will they come, and will they know anything about AIDS? Skilled nursing care is surely anticipated. From whence will it come? Direct and ancillary support services are equally remote. . . .

Our citizens are understandably alarmed by the contagion factor. We should also be concerned with the quality of treatment the patients will receive in Highland County. How will it compare with the responsive care which they now have available by people with experience in the field of AIDS?

Of equal concern is the commitment of the county to a proposal which conceivably could become a burden and an embarrassment. Dr. Kübler-Ross states that she will not ask for any reimbursement for taking these children in. Does this mean she will not apply for any federal or state grants? Will her services qualify for payment through Medicare/Medicaid or some other third party, or will she be dependent on contributions? How are the victims now being supported and will that financing be transferrable to Highland County and the Commonwealth of Virginia? Who will pay for the transportation by air or rescue squad in case of an emergency? If a child should die, who pays the burial expenses? . . .

H. W.
McDowell, Virginia

September 29, 1985

Editor:

I am discouraged by the way Dr. Kübler-Ross announced her plans for an AIDS center. She might have told her neighbors before she told the networks.

Still, I do support those plans.

One day, soon, the AIDS panic will subside. When it does, what will we in Highland want to say for ourselves?

Despite the real difficulties and our fear, we sought to comfort helpless, dying children.

G. H.
Williamsville, Virginia

September 30, 1985

Editor:

My husband and I have been raising sheep in Highland County for the past fifteen years and this is one of the few times I feel the county has been presented with a real moral dilemma. There is no question that AIDS is a terrifying disease because to date it has been 100 percent fatal.

I have no quarrel with anyone who questions the implementation of Elisabeth Kübler-Ross's AIDS center for children. There are intelligent and reasonable questions to be asked, questions concerning the possible contact of these children with the community (it was stated, however, in *The Recorder* that "Children would be kept on the premises through all stages of the disease"), with any potential expense which might be borne by the county to support this facility, questions neighbors might legitimately ask, such as how waste material which could contain contaminating substances (blood) would be disposed of— through drainage, a septic system, etcetera.

What disturbs me is not that people are asking

serious questions about the proposed AIDS center, but that people are opposing it before Dr. Kübler-Ross has had a chance to answer all the questions the residents of our county might ask. I believe it is the responsibility of each of us, if we intend to take a stand either way on this issue, to be as well informed as possible, to attend Dr. Kübler-Ross's public meeting October 9, and to pose well thought out questions. I, for one, will be both personally troubled and embarrassed for the county if we are not fair-minded and civil during the discussions.

But this works both ways. While it might have been wiser for Dr. Kübler-Ross to have held an AIDS discussion with Highland County residents prior to her announcement to the media, at this point she had an obligation to be accessible, informative, and patient with all questions raised. . . .

One could hardly argue with the fact that Elisabeth Kübler-Ross has been a person who has dedicated her life to helping others. Several years ago I heard her talk on a PBS special about the work she was doing with children dying of cancer. I was deeply touched by her wisdom and compassion and by her special gift for helping these children accept their imminent deaths.

Given the uncertainty of AIDS, it is true that not many counties in the U.S. would welcome such a center without reservations. But with joint cooperation, this issue may represent an opportunity and a challenge for our county and Dr. Kübler-Ross to accomplish something few others would undertake.

A. W.
Headwaters, Virginia

September 30, 1985

Editor:

As far as I know, not a single case of AIDS has been found among our Highland people.

Have you stopped to consider what effect this center will have on our county? The taxes will go up drastically as soon as they begin operation, especially if there are any school-aged children. They will demand educational classes and the county will have to comply.

The land values will go down, as people who were expecting to come to our county to live will go elsewhere. And any chance of economic growth will go out the window.

Why come to a sparsely populated area. Why not near a metropolitan area where medical aid is readily available, and the area is much more able to handle the extra cost that such a program will engender?

Where are the doctors and nurses to come from? What will this facility eventually become? We may end up with the adult AIDS victims too.

If I remember correctly, when this land was bought, it was to be a training center to train people in how to care for terminally ill people, and a hospice for terminally ill elderly people. If not stated specifically, it was intimated that this was the actual goal. What had happened to that?

It seems to me that this whole project was started under false pretenses. Who knows just what will happen if our supervisors allow this to come into our county.

I do not want to see my children, grandchildren,

and all our Highland people burdened with something they do not deserve, do you? Are we to become a dumping ground for what more affluent areas don't want?

I strongly urge you to talk to our supervisors and to attend the October meeting.

Highlanders! Stand up and be counted.

L. B.

October 7, 1985

Editor:

As a former resident of Highland County, and having friends and relatives there, I have been following with great interest the letters concerning the proposed AIDS center. I wrote to Dr. Kübler-Ross, telling her of my feelings concerning the center. As of this date, I have received no reply—and I expect none.

After reading an article in the Parkersburg (West Virginia) *News,* it really started me wondering. Just what does the good doctor really have in mind? Quoting the article, ". . . they were also stirred to action by a comment made last June in Boston by Dr. Kübler-Ross, a noted authority on death and dying. Kübler-Ross said that 'any hospice which failed to accept an AIDS patient ought to be closed,' DiTullio said."

What part of her plans has she shared with others outside Highland County that she hasn't shared with our local people? The article, allegedly quoting her, tells me that she would accept anyone, regardless of age or condition, if she opens the AIDS center.

Part of my feelings on [this] matter has already been covered by F. P., J. T., and L. B., so I will state the second part, as an outsider who has friends and relatives in Highland. This is regarding the consequences of fear. It is not true, in this case, that "We have nothing to fear but fear itself."

I feel Highland County can be ruined from the fear outside Highland, as well as inside. Highland County depends on the trade from tourists, from outsiders attending Maple Festivals, fall festivals, and county fairs, people who come to see your beautiful mountains, enjoy the warmth of your people, and to see and buy your handicrafts. If you have this proposed center there, everyone will be afraid and business will suffer, not only in Highland itself, but as far north as Franklin and as far west as Bartow. . . .

Why should Highland bear the burden of financial responsibility and the many other burdens this proposed center would impose upon her people? Speaking of the Christian ideal, isn't it applicable to both sides?

If these children are being sent here to die, what about the children themselves, hundreds of miles from their parents. No matter how lovingly cared for, a child who loves and looks to its parents for love and security, dies alone if its parents aren't there. Will Highlanders stand up and be counted? Who would send their desperately ill children hundreds of miles to die among strangers, where they cannot be adequately cared for? You won't find any Highlander who would be so unloving and cruel.

The years my children and I spent in Highland County were loving ones. During the time of my husband's illness and death, and following that, my two serious operations, I really couldn't have made it through if it hadn't been for the help and caring of my Highland neighbors, who rallied round. They are caring people. They have the right to say no to a situation that could endanger their children and grandchildren, when an outsider could wipe out, within a short time, what their forebears had built through many generations.

H. H.
Coolville, Ohio

October 16, 1985

Editor:

I have been watching the controversy regarding Dr. Kübler-Ross's proposal to care for infants and young children who are AIDS victims. Some of the facts are generally agreed on. The children are very young. They are unwanted elsewhere. They will die within two years of acquiring the disease through no fault of their own. The proposed site is remote from residential areas.

While much remains unknown about AIDS, it is clear at this point that exposure to body fluids of a victim is necessary for transmission of the disease. Dr. Kübler-Ross has agreed to isolate these children from the community at large, and to use recommended medical procedures as appropriate.

119

Since Highland County is such a Christian area, and since Jesus has set the precedent by working with lepers, one would expect the citizens of Highland County to take pity on these poor children. One would be wrong. Apparently what the Highland folk hear on Sunday has little to do with their behavior during the week.

These innocent and unfortunate children have had a little lamp of hope lit by Dr. Kübler-Ross. Now the uncharitable hypocrites of Highland County are doing their best to blow it out. Maybe they've never heard of charity or of "doing unto others." More likely, they follow their religious beliefs only when their beliefs happen to meet their own selfish ends.

E. W.
Staunton, Virginia

Editor:

In regard to Mr. E. W.'s letter of October 16, I want to point out to him that the people in Highland County do have great respect and pity for the children who have AIDS. But we also have much concern and pity for our own children, as well as our adults who might be affected and ill from AIDS, if we let Dr. Ross unload AIDS in our community.

Most residents of Highland County don't want to see our county become a dump site for AIDS. I don't know what business it is of Mr. W.'s what we do in Highland County. If Mr. W. wants an AIDS center for Dr. Ross, why doesn't he get it somewhere where he could be close to it? He sure needs to be there.

This is a worldwide problem. Why bring it to Highland County? If we are all uncharitable hypocrites in Highland County, I don't believe it is a good place for a center like this or Dr. Ross either.

I don't know what Mr. W. calls himself, but I am sure he is not a hypocrite. A hypocrite would have more respect than to write a letter like this to the people of his neighboring county. I don't believe he knows anything about hypocrisy or Christianity either. Mr. W., please don't judge the people in Highland County by your own self.

M. S.
Monterey, Virginia

October 15, 1985

Editor:

I have been reading everything I can find on Elisabeth Kübler-Ross center in Highland County and her plan for treating AIDS patients, and I can tell you without reservation that all I feel is shock. Dr. Kübler-Ross, how could you do this to a community so beautiful, so pure and unspoiled? There is no place in the East so beautiful, and still you chose to bring the most dread disease of our century into its midst.

Anyone who opposes this plan is hysterical. Don't make the people of this area feel that they are less Christian if they speak out. Why are these AIDS patients being taken from the inner city where the disease is more prevalent and the hospitals more prepared to deal with it, as they have done for some time?

Why do some doctors in our area seem to be so sure of their knowledge of AIDS, and the U.S. Centers for Disease Control in Atlanta is proceding with extreme caution?

Let's get back to basics. Common sense and caution are the key words here. If it's compassion you feel, use your compassion on a community you are tearing apart, people living in an environment of clean, simple living that has been fought for and protected by the forefathers. Elisabeth, there are two sides to every coin.

M. N.
West Augusta, Virginia

October 15, 1985

Editor:

I believe that Dr. Kübler-Ross has a right to build a privately funded center for abandoned babies with AIDS on her own land in Headwaters if it does not pose any substantial health risk or zoning problems. I also believe that county residents and landowners have a right to receive answers to their concerns about health risks. What I cannot support is the view that the center should be stopped whether or not it poses any real health threat.

Public image can be a very shallow thing that judges from outside appearances only. I personally think it's unlikely that fear of AIDS will keep many (if any) tourists away from such a beautiful place as

Highland; it doesn't seem to have kept anyone away from the big cities where it's more prevalent.

I agree with Dr. Babb, who stated at the public meeting on October 9 that the county will [be] hurt far worse by refusing the center. But, even if I'm wrong, is this fear of image a good moral reason for preventing Dr. Kübler-Ross from using her land as her conscience dictates?

What if one of our children here in Highland had the terrible misfortune to contract the AIDS virus through a blood transfusion; would we want that child to come home as soon as the doctors advised, or would we worry about the reputation of the county and prefer to have that child stay? I cannot imagine that people in Highland would close their doors in such an instance.

Whether or not Dr. Kübler-Ross is allowed to proceed with her plans now rests with the State Health Department, the county zoning board, and the board of supervisors, It is very important that these public officials are allowed to focus on the legitimate issues of health and zoning and not pressured by fears of bad image.

P. S.
Monterey, Virginia

October 20, 1985

Editor:

It had been inferred that helping Kübler-Ross care for AIDS victims is the godly, caring thing to do and that a true Christian would support such a thing.

Kübler-Ross aligns herself with Jesus, saying, "He never turned away lepers or the sick." But what is she doing for the dying and sick? Is she healing them or leading them to Christ? When asked at the meeting in Monterey if she taught them to die in Jesus Christ, she did not answer. Her only reply was, "I'm a Christian." Jesus Christ never professed reincarnation. Hitler claimed to be a Christian.

Is Kübler-Ross a follower of Christ? If not, the churches should not support her or wish [her] Godspeed, lest they themselves help the damnation of innocent souls. She was quoted last year on a television interview with theologians as saying the Bible supports reincarnation.

This county does not have the facilities to provide for these children adequately. Kübler-Ross's intentions are not clear. Most importantly, she studies death and dying to further her own beliefs in reincarnation. Although she may or may not be sincere, her teachings are false, against God's word, and certainly doesn't help the victims. It only furthers the deception. We as Christians should not accept condemnation in any respect for not helping her.

J. C.
McDowell, Virginia

October 21, 1985

Editor:

How do these liberal politicians get off telling employers not hiring AIDS victims is an act of discrimination as is the case in Los Angeles? Who gives them the right to allow these victims to infect others which can and most likely will happen if they are allowed to deal with the public in the forms of food, public health services, etcetera?

Who suffers when businesses lose customers as a result? Not just the AIDS victim but the business. Who wants to eat at a place where food is handled by these victims, for instance? I wouldn't! So not hiring them is not discrimination, but exercising plain common sense. I'm not saying they shouldn't be hired for some jobs, but when there's a chance someone else may become infected as a result of their work, then they shouldn't be hired.

If liberals and politicians really want to do something to get rid of AIDS, they should start with the gays and their activities. Most sane people know homosexuality is indecent, immoral, and unethical. They're not a special species. They are just males and females that are supposed to have the same rights as we do—no more, no less. So why not outlaw it? No, they'd rather condone this and prosecute someone trying to protect their interests. They're concerned too much about the legalities and formalities rather than the destruction of it.

If they were victims of cholera, they'd be quarantined; if victims of leporosy, they used to be sent to leper colonies and considered as outcasts. So why not do something to protect the public against AIDS? It's just as deadly.

The victims I feel sorry for are the ones that have or will contract the disease by no fault of their own.

If you are concerned, write your congressman

and tell him it's time they did more about it. We have the right to be protected, too!

J. G.
Greenville, Virginia

October 22, 1985

Editor:

As usual when a controversial issue confronts this area, the zealots and fanatics have come creeping out of the woodwork hurling invective and abuse. Mr. E. W., I will not sit still for being called an "uncharitable hypocrite," nor can I allow my neighbors to be likewise insulted.

To most Highland residents with whom I have talked (and believe me the AIDS center and Dr. Kübler-Ross are hot topics), the opposition is not to "taking pity on these poor children." We are not any more afraid of AIDS than we are of cancer or polio (or leprosy). No, Mr. E. W., what concerns us about Dr. Kübler-Ross's plan is her lack of planning.

She does not now have the proper facilities to provide these children with the care they will require, and she cannot or will not show concrete evidence that proper facilities are in the works. Children don't die of AIDS, they die of flu or pneumonia or any number of other communicable diseases that their little bodies can't fight off because AIDS has destroyed their immunologic systems. To give them proper care, they need to be in a facility that can provide isolation from disease, excellent treatment for those they do contract, and proximity to the intensive research now mobilizing in search of a cure.

Dr. Kübler-Ross has not been able to prove to the residents of Highland County that she can provide proper facilities, competent health care personnel, or adequate transportation for these children. The only thing she has shown so far is a penchant for attracting publicity and an appalling lack of regard for her neighbors. The first inkling most of us had of her plans was when we saw it on the evening news and in the newspapers. The way she has handled this campaign to date has caused many Highland residents to doubt her motives. . . .

B. C.
McDowell, Virginia

October 23, 1985

Editor:

This letter is in response to the letter written Wednesday October 16, by E. W.

Mr. E. W., how can you call people hypocrites whom you don't know? We are not hypocrites, just people who are only trying to protect their interests and heritage that was left them by their forefathers.

The Bible says, "Judge not, lest ye be judged." Well, who gave you the right to judge the people in Highland County? One old saying I've always heard is "It takes one to know one."

As there are no known cases of AIDS in High-

127

land, why should we chance bringing it into our community? If Mr. E. W. is so righteous and supportive of this center, why doesn't he just invite Dr. Kübler-Ross to bring these children into his home and use it for the center? There is a hospital in Staunton. I'm sure his neighbors wouldn't think too much of that.

Sure, I, like the other people here, feel sorry for these children, but most of the cases are in the bigger cities where there are bigger hospitals and better facilities to handle these cases. Why take children three hundred to three thousand miles to a place so isolated where there is no hospital within forty miles? I don't feel that this issue has anything to do with being a Christian to get the center, but people's lives and how this will affect them and the best for the community.

Highland County has been my home all my life and I for one am against the AIDS center in our county. I think Mr. E. W. had better do some soul searching and not judge other people.

R. C.
Monterey, Virginia

October 23, 1985

Editor:

In regard to E. W.'s letter, it is very apparent he doesn't know much about what he is running off at the mouth about. It seems he is more than a hypocrite.

First off, it (the proposed AIDS center) is not remote from residential areas and if he is so concerned we suggest that Dr. Kübler-Ross build a center in his back yard and see how loud he yells.

K. T.
Staunton, Virginia

October 23, 1985

Editor:

We are replying to Mr. E. W.'s letter in the October 16 issue regarding the AIDS center in Highland County.

We do not feel that we should be called hypocrites because we are opposed to the AIDS center. In the Bible it says, "Judge not that ye not be judged."

If Ms. Kübler-Ross is not able to establish the AIDS center in Highland County, it would be practical for her to establish it in Staunton.

Staunton is actually a better location for the center because of the modern hospital facilities which the children could be near.

Since there is little known on the AIDS subject, and no known cure, we firmly believe that being opposed to the AIDS center in Highland County is common sense.

N. E.
W. R.
Doe Hill, Virginia

October 23, 1985

Editor:

Recently we moved from Highland County to Fairfax for financial reasons. Our dream is to move back to Highland with our small children and raise our family there.

I have never seen a community more filled with loving, giving people than Highland. We moved there, newcomers, with no friends or relatives. We left reluctantly and sadly. We constantly miss the caring, friendly people.

Don't let anyone tell you that Highland people are ignorant or running scared. When it comes to AIDS, nobody knows for sure and nobody can promise anything. It's not blind fear that is in the minds of Highlanders, but careful, thoughtful deliberation. Let me assure you, in this highly educated, high income Fairfax County, with doctors and hospitals abounding (and certainly more AIDS victims), there is no way the citizens would allow an AIDS treatment center to be built. Not because of hate or demonic spirits, but because of a natural instinct to protect home and family.

It is not un-Christian or ignorant to disagree with Kübler-Ross. As residents you have a right to be informed and to protect Highland County. You should expect your elected officials to respond to your wishes and not allow this center to be built. As Christians you have a command to protect your families. Then to pray, for unfortunate victims of AIDS, and for the enlightenment of Kübler-Ross and her followers. Don't let her make you defensive because she mentions Jesus. God was in Highland County and His work was being done there long before this proposed AIDS center and He will be there long after it is forgotten.

R. D.
Fairfax, Virginia

October 24, 1985

Editor:

I read with dismay of the opposition of Highland County residents to a proposed home for child AIDS victims.

They wanted total assurance from Dr. Kübler-Ross that they would not contract the disease. What utter folly!

Have any of us assurance that we won't be hit by an automobile as we cross the street, or even that we won't die of a heart attack before the end of this day? What of the cigarettes many smoke and the food we eat that contains chemicals?

One has but to read Matthew 24 to see that Jesus predicted famine, earthquakes, and pestilences in the last days. Is not AIDS a pestilence?

The physician from Charlottesville was quoted as saying this disease is spread by adults. He did not say children. True, this disease is a dreadful one and people wish to protect their own children, but think for a moment of the little ones who already have this disease and have been abandoned.

God has promised to take care of his own. Perhaps we would all do well to read Matthew 5–7 and endeavor to make these words of Jesus our standard.

B. L.
Boones Mill, Virginia

October 24, 1985

Editor:

This is in response to Mr. E. W.'s unjust attack on Highland people in a recent issue of your paper and to Dr. Elisabeth Kübler-Ross's proposed AIDS center.

When Jesus was tempted by the devil he responded with scripture. To Mr. E. W., I quote Matthew 7, "Judge not that ye be not judged. Why beholdest thou the mote that is in thy brother's eye, but considerest not the beam that is in thine own eye? Thou hypocrite. . . ."

Does Dr. Kübler-Ross believe that removing these children from their present abode (where they are) provided with food, clothing, shelter, and medication serves any real purpose? She indicated she wants to hold them, provide a toy for them and watch them die. Are these her ideas of good works? Ephesians 2 tells us, "For it is by the grace of God ye are saved, and not of good works."

One need only turn on TV to see the thousands who are dying from lack of food and water and are naked and need medication. Where is her love and compassion for these? . . .

I am proud of our county and the people who have devoted a lifetime of hard work in helping the county be what it is today. I am not implying that we are indestructible, but with God's help we press on to the high calling of God in Christ Jesus.

R. K.
Monterey, Virginia

October 24, 1985

Editor:

In response to Mr. E. W.'s letter, I wish to defend the people of Highland County in their fight against the proposed AIDS center.

Being a nonresident landowner of Highland County, and in contact with many of the residents, I have found the statement that they are uncharitable hypocrites to be unfounded and incorrect.

The liberal thinking and attitude of Mr. E. W. speaks for itself. Use of the remote area of Highland County as a guinea pig is all right, but certainly not here in Staunton or other residential areas.

It would seem to me that they are fighting not against the children but against AIDS which is proven to be spead by homosexuals, bisexuals, etcetera, which Dr. Kübler-Ross certainly has not guaranteed will not be kept at the proposed AIDS center.

S. B.
Mount Sidney, Virginia

October 24, 1985

Editor:

E. W.'s letter to the editor October 16 shows how little he knows about that of which he speaks.

I would ask where he gets his information and his right to criticize the religion of Highland County people? Before E. W. becomes judge and jury of Highland County people's religion, he should know that each individual's religion is between that individual and his God. That is none of E. W.'s concern.

"Hypocrite" and "uncharitable" seem to be favorite words in his vocabulary. I've been taught that name-calling is beneath the dignity of anyone.

I wonder if E. W. would like to take unfortunate AIDS children and hover them under his charitable wings?

It is not one's place to judge another because the judgment is most often incorrect and unfair.

M. R.
Monterey, Virginia

October 27, 1985

Editor:

"Infuriated" mildly describes the way I felt after reading E. W.'s letter in a recent issue of your newspaper regarding the people of Highland County and Dr. Kübler-Ross's desire to establish a facility for the care of very young AIDS victims.

It pleases me that some good Highlanders have taken the time to respond, both through your newspaper and by telephone.

Being born and reared in Highland County, I am proud to be a Highlander. The years I did not live in Highland, E. W., his parents, and brother were our across-the-street neighbors. I don't know how many Highlanders E. may be acquainted with, other than the good Highland farmers who delivered fresh eggs to the W. family many, many years.

I believe in freedom of speech, but not when it is used to accuse and belittle as E. W. did to our citizens, who in my opinion, are most compassionate and caring.

It is my wish that E. W. will let the "heat" (his word) that he is receiving teach him a lesson not to stick his nose and neck in matters not concerning him. If the proposed Kübler-Ross AIDS facility were being built in Staunton, E. W. would be the first to start jumping up and down and complaining.

G. S.
McDowell, Virginia

November 8, 1985

Editor:

I have been waiting for a Christian letter from Highland County in support of the attempt of Dr. Elisabeth Kübler-Ross to give AIDS victims the love and care these innocent children need. But all I've seen so far is criticism for her for wanting to do her good works in Highland County, and criticism of E. W. for supporting Kübler-Ross and the AIDS center and calling people a name they deserve.

One letter criticized Kübler-Ross because "she

indicated she wants to hold them, provide a toy for them," and care for them till they die. "Are these her ideas of good works?" the writer said. She wants Kübler-Ross to forget AIDS victims and help "the thousands who are dying from lack of food and water."

Maybe Highland people show their Christianity by helping the hungry. But why are they criticizing Kübler-Ross for her attempt to do good works?

It's a big world. And there's plenty of good works for the Lord's people to do. But all of us don't have the same job. Christians have always taken in children no one wants to help. Highland County Christians should be proud they have someone there who is willing to love and care for children most people are afraid to help.

When so-called Christians tell Kübler-Ross to go somewhere else and do her good works, and stop her from caring for helpless AIDS victims in their county, aren't they hypocrites? What's more hypocritical than telling her to do her good works in Staunton or any place except a county that doesn't belong to God but to them?

The Earth is the Lord's—all of it—including Highland County.

K. C.
Greenville, Virginia

December 3, 1985

Editor:

I have read several articles about the intention of Dr. Kübler-Ross to open a home for deserted AIDS children. With astonishment I learn that there is great opposition in the community against this prospect.

Being a European and knowing Dr. Kübler-Ross personally, I think many places in the old country would be proud and thankful if she had chosen one of our communities to help those children who are in urgent need of love, care, and understanding.

Some people are afraid. Of what? Science has found under what conditions that disease can be spread.

In my hand is a dollar bill with the motto "In God We Trust." Did this wonderful country of America become big by being chicken? Certainly not. But if people really trust in God, they must know that their life span lies within His fatherly hands, and man cannot add a single day to it. So why be afraid?

I understand that not everyone can provide a home for outcasts, disabled, crippled, and sick people. And not everyone wants to. There are just a few people who devote their lives to benefit others. But I cannot comprehend people who try to prevent a person like Dr. Kübler-Ross from doing what has to be done.

In my few weeks in Lynchburg, I have met so many friendly people with so much kindness that I am sure those people in the mountains are much the same and will finally accept those children in their neighborhood.

S. F.
Lynchburg, Virginia

Chapter 6

Finding a Way

We continue to farm, to raise food, to can and preserve, and we welcome everybody who inquires seriously about our work and workshops. Thousands of people who want to rid themselves of their fears and to take care of their unfinished business so they can go on living and becoming more whole, continue to sign up for these workshops. The thousands of letters received regularly testify to the effectiveness of those workshops, some of which, we hope, we will be able to offer at our own center, adjacent to the farm.

The nationally viewed Monterey meeting resulted in another onslaught of mail, 95 percent of which was not only in our favor, but with bits and pieces of support, advice, and offers of help. Volunteers started to appear from all over the country. At the time of this writing, we have twelve volunteers who assist us in gardening, farming, bringing in the hay, construction work on the center, and knitting for needy children. A neighbor brought in and donated a knitting machine. The upstairs of my house looks like a storehouse with wools, dolls, and stuffed animals for those children. At the same time, people started to write from other countries. An older lady who sat lonely and unsatisfied with her empty life suddenly started to leave her apartment in Canada. She discovered that she was able to buy old dolls for fifty cents apiece in local flea markets. She spent her mornings shopping for such treasures, and her afternoons and evenings sewing outfits and knitting clothing for those dolls. A package arrived shortly before Christmas; sewn into an old bedsheet was a gift of the best-dressed dolls, which would be a delight for many of these children!

A middle-aged woman from North Carolina approached me with wet eyes at the end of a five-day workshop and confessed that the week changed her entire life and outlook. She said that her brother was a Baptist minister and she was warned by him that she might be in the company of dying patients, including AIDS patients, if she attended my workshop. She came with great trepidations and doubts. When, by the middle of the week, she was able to get in touch with her own unfinished business and truly let go of her fears, she felt a great relief with an upsurge of tremendous compassion and love for her fellow man. When she said good-bye to me, she shook my hand and gave me a big hug, and said, "You know, we were never able to hug anybody. It was construed as immoral. And imagine, today I hugged an AIDS patient and I was not the least bit hesitant about it. In fact, I loved it and I am proud of myself."

I have seen other such transformations. A woman originally signed up for the workshop to increase her skills as a hospice volunteer. During the course of the week, she became aware of her very inhibiting and restrictive childhood. She increasingly allowed herself to feel her own feelings rather than just to smile when "others expected her to smile," and she finally dropped her "front," the mask that she wore all her life. In fact, we discovered a very genuinely warm and joyful woman, full of humor and compassion—a distinct difference from the stiff, uptight person she had been on the first day. Hesitantly at first, then with obvious pleasure, she joined in the sharing of the many who dealt with similar unnatural upbringings and started to enjoy hugging and laughing with her roommates and other participants.

It has been one year since the conception of the idea about an AIDS baby hospice on my farm. It has become clear that this community is not about to give us a rezoning of a small piece of my own farmland. To fight against such fear and negativity is only adding to the resistance and the hostility. We learned a long time ago, and continue to teach the fact, that negativity can only survive on negativity. This does not mean that we have given up the idea. We will, naturally, have hospices for children, including AIDS babies and toddlers. Once I gave up the idea of having such a place of love and peace and healing on my own land, I decided to look for other acceptable alternatives. We keep our 25,000 supporters nationwide informed about our plans, knowing that our newsletter is also widely read in our own community, where it is always available at our local Headwaters post office.

I used my enormous mail resources (we receive 250,000 pieces of mail a year), as well as the newsletter, to inquire about families who would be willing to become foster parents to AIDS babies. Many parents called up and inquired about the requirements for such an undertaking. They had a million questions and I answered them as best I could. I purposely painted a dark picture should they make such a commitment. I told them that these children were very susceptible to all sorts of infections, parasites, and fungi. They would often have diarrhea and/or throw up. They might cry incessantly and need to be carried around. Their own children might be ostracized in school and not allowed to visit their playmates in their homes any longer. I even brought up the idea that the local school board might question their children's right to attend the public school once it was known that they housed a child with AIDS.

I insisted that all these aspects had to be discussed with all members of the family, including children and grandparents. I even suggested that their commitment was for a lifetime, not just for a few months or a year. Should a successful treatment be found and these children survive, the foster parents would then be responsible for the children's education, as if they were one of their own. Only if *all* family members agreed to take on such a patient would I start the procedures.

Parents, whose children had died years ago, and whom I had helped in their time of need, offered to sponsor a child financially. People who lived on their marginal Social Security started to send five dollars a month "for the children." I made it clear to all potential foster parents that they should take these children without payment if at all possible. It had to be a gift of unconditional love, and their rewards would be far greater than monetary compensation. I emphasized that all of our work with dying

141

patients for the last twenty years had been free of charge, and this was the only way to truly serve. I reminded them that God always provides for our needs and He would do the same for all of those who are willing to help their brothers and sisters in need. It was beautiful for me to see the response. Not one family requested "a white child," or said, "Please don't give me a Haitian child." They, truly, were ready to practice what we were supposed to have learned for two thousand years—and so many still have a hard time learning.

While my home became an informal foster care agency and the already-busy telephone did not stop ringing, I had to continue with my scheduled lectures and workshops. My office staff did the best they could in my absence, and volunteers continued to take care of my farm. More and more adult AIDS patients had the courage to attend my workshops, and they gained a great deal from them. There were always one or two reluctant participants who did not want to share the same bedroom or dining room table with those patients, but they soon were able to get in touch with their fears and let go of them.

There was never any pressure put on the participants, and they were free to leave the workshop if it became too threatening for them. We had fewer participants leave the workshops after the inclusion of AIDS patients than all the ten years before! In the fall of 1985 we received the first desperate phone calls from social workers around the country asking for assistance in the placement of AIDS babies. They were familiar with my work with dying children and knew me as a founding member of the Children's Hospice International, Inc. Many had attended my lectures or workshops. The occurrence of AIDS among small children was obviously on the rise.

142

While there were more and more reported cases of hemophiliacs who were suddenly showing symptoms of AIDS, the social workers were concerned with the increase in the number of babies that started to show up who were not hemophiliacs. These were children of apparently healthy young women, yet they were showing all the signs of having defective immune systems.

Some of them were children of prostitutes and/or drug users. Once the diagnosis of PAID (pediatric AIDS) was confirmed, the life expectancy of these often very sick and always very vulnerable children was very short. Many of the IV drug-using and often single mothers were financially, emotionally, and physically unable to take care of them. Some simply dropped them in hospitals, never to visit them again. Some moved away and were unreachable when a crisis occurred and the hospital staff needed to contact them. Thus, they were left in hospital rooms with nursing staffs around the clock but without any permanent familiar faces. When they came out of their medical crisis, they were not discharged to a family or a less institutional environment. They often spent months and months in the same hospital rooms, never able to play with other children, or run around in a garden, or play with pets. They never were taken out into the sunshine, to toy shops or parks. There were no foster families who were available to take them in between hospitalizations, and so they were institutionalized until they died.

Needless to say, there were exceptions. We, naturally, were only called when a caring social worker "just couldn't handle it anymore." There were people in New York, New Jersey, and Massachusetts who took some of these children, but they were the great exceptions rather than the rule.

143

By the late fall of 1985, I was informed that there were nearly a hundred of these children in institutions that really did not need to spend the rest of their lives in hospitals. All this information was given to me rather secretively out of fear that the hospital could hear about it and the case worker would be fired.

In January 1986, I had compiled a remarkable list of potential foster families and called the hospitals that appeared to have a great number of these children. I expected to get an enthusiastic response, but instead, in each case, I got a real runaround. The person in charge was either "on vacation" or "out of the office." After a half dozen phone calls, I wrote letters. No one wrote back. In February I called again. After a similar runaround at one hospital I finally asked to speak with the supervisor. The woman I spoke with advised me to "just forget it." It was then that I realized that the issue was far greater than I had bargained for. One social worker with whom I spoke was very interested in finding out how I was able to find so many caring families who were willing to take on such a burden. I told her it might seem like a burden to her, but to those families it was a blessing that brought the whole family closer together and allowed them to share an incredible amount of love. She was incredulous and hung up on me!

In the early spring (again in-between travels and just after returning from New Zealand and Australia, where the AIDS epidemic was just starting to become known), I decided it was time to go to some of the big cities of the East Coast. I wanted to visit some of the well-known centers and talk to the physicians in charge. And I hoped to visit some of these children and to evaluate how we could effectively help the patients and the staff. But once again

144

I got nowhere. One physician promised to call me back "by 10 P.M." He never called back. After several attempts to meet with him, he told me that he was too busy to see me at the hospital, but he would not mind coming to see me at my hotel in New York. I checked into the hotel where I had told him I would be staying, but he never came to see me. (I thought it strange that someone was too busy to see me at the hospital but would be able to make a rather lengthy trip to Manhattan. Was that to keep me away from his place of work?!) I used that trip, and that opportunity, to visit with the newly elected cardinal of the Episcopal church, who was more than generous and cordial with his time and interest. I left his office reassured of the support of his church, and feeling a bit more confident about the sad role of many churches in the area of AIDS.

By now I had spent a great deal of time and energy finding suitable places for these "unwanted" AIDS babies, and one thing had become clear to me: While there were a few cases and social workers who pleaded for changes in policy, they all sounded intimidated or rather paranoid in handling and discussing the problems with these children.

Politics and money apparently started to contaminate the picture, and I felt as if I were putting my hands into a wasps' nest once again—the story of my life!

I was aware of a Haitian child who had been kept in the hospital on the East Coast and, according to a case worker, at $1,000 a day the hospital had "no intentions of giving this child to a foster family." Naturally, with money coming into a hospital in these amounts, an administrator

145

would be a fool to release such a child to a foster family, especially if the family were willing to take the child in at no cost at all. This seemed to shed some light on the secondary gains and interest, aside from the benefits of doing research, on these unclaimed children, who do not have an advocate to present their rights.

What about the money that would be available for research, what would happen to that extra source of funding, if all these children were taken away and placed in foster homes? What about the scientific data that would stop being available if these babies and toddlers were discharged the minute they no longer required any further hospitalization until their next bout of life-threatening infections?

I decided to head for the "big cities" on the East Coast a second time and take a personal look. All these hospitals know me well from my work with dying patients, and many had asked repeatedly for lectures and in-service seminars for their doctors and health-care staff. So I believed I'd have no problem going there myself and taking a look at the problems the staff and the patients and their families might face in view of this new and not-yet-really-understood disease.

The reality proved to be very different from my expectations! I had made arrangements for a friend to pick me up at the airport in order to have some time to talk. Instead, a woman physician came, saying my friend was unavailable to see me. I thought that strange, as I had talked with her on the phone the night before and everything had been arranged. I was received at the hospital elevator by a number of people and was escorted to an office where those staff members who were willing to see me were assembled. It was a strange and stiff meeting. I

146

told them of my work and interest in children and others with AIDS, my hopes to be of help and assistance to the staff, and my workshops with both staff and patients. The group seemed very defensive, claimed to have only one child with AIDS at the present, and showed no enthusiasm for the list of twenty-seven foster-home families I had collected in the interim.

I was allowed to accompany the head nurse to see the two-year-old child who had never been visited by her mother. The latter apparently blamed her husband for the child's illness and left it up to the father to visit her occasionally. With no money and little conversation with a child who never learned to speak, those visits were rare and few indeed. The hospital room looked like any child's room, with toys and stuffed animals and a caring nurse who was obviously attached to the child. She brought out a tricycle and allowed her to scoot around the hospital hallway. Across the hall were the other pediatric beds with sick children covered by bedsheets or hidden behind oxygen tents, parents sitting at their bedsides—oblivious to the happily scooting around child with AIDS who was rarely ever visited by her next of kin.

Why was this child kept here for eight months when the same hospital had had my list of volunteer families for several months? Why is so much money spent on a two-year-old who did not require acute hospital care and did not have a family to take her home? Sure, this baby was admitted to the hospital in an emaciated state and very poor health, but that was months ago!

I felt as if I had just opened a Pandora's box as the questions raced through my mind. Where was the money coming from to pay for a child who should have been discharged months ago? At a thousand dollars a day, the taxpayers were losing a fortune. But totally aside from financial considerations, these children needed a healthy environment, not a pediatric unit where other sick children were only an arm's length away.

These children also need a more permanent love object, not constantly shifting nurses no matter how much some of them become attached to these babies and toddlers. They need sunshine and a garden and playmates, and they have to be allowed to see and touch a flower and watch a butterfly in flight!

Chapter 7

Women and AIDS

Mothers of AIDS children and women with AIDS must not be neglected either. Women with AIDS have a hard time, not only in facing the dread disease and all its consequences, but, worst of all, the dreadful and almost uniform rejection and isolation. A two-year-old child has, at least, the parents and/or care-giver and may receive less direct hostility from her environment. A woman, however, will return to her apartment after she has been diagnosed and discharged only to discover that her old friends stop visiting, refuse to see her—even stop calling.

Bonny was one of those who had to go through this ordeal and in her own words had "never felt so utterly alone in the world." Had it not been for her two cats, who seemed to become even more affectionate and closer to her, she does not know what would have happened to her. Raised in Germany and always full of life, fun, and a delight to be around, she found herself more and more withdrawn, spending days at home watching TV or staring into space. She used to love her work, but at thirty-three, she suddenly felt like a lonely old woman "forgotten by the world." She contracted her disease years ago when she was engaged to a man who had been a heavy drug user. The relationship ended and for her it was a story of the past. "Of the past" until she became more and more fatigued, more and more prone to infection, she lost a lot of weight and while in the hospital for a recurrent pneumonia, the diagnosis of AIDS was verified.

In the fall of 1982, Bonny's life changed in such a way that she started to make arrangements for her funeral; she even bought an urn for her ashes. It would take two more years before she finally knew why her life seemed to go downhill much too rapidly for such a young woman. It was after reading several newspaper articles that she began to suspect what she might be suffering from. She signed herself into the hospital. Her first reaction was one of great relief. It was the "not knowing," the uncertainty, that almost killed her. Now, at least, she knew where she stood. Why did the other doctors wait so long to share what they always suspected? It was the day-to-day existence that she had to face now as a woman with AIDS. Friends refused to come, they were afraid to sit at the same kitchen table with her as they had done for so many years. They were afraid to touch her hand, and they avoided her when she ran into one of them at the street corner. They avoided her looks. A young couple who had befriended her and visited many times before the diagnosis was made was evicted from the building by another couple who feared that their children might catch the disease. Bonny's life shrank to a lonely existence in her apartment with a silent telephone and a house bell that never rang.

A former workshop participant heard about her and called her up. She invited Bonny to mobilize all her strength and pack a bag, she would pick her up the next day and drive her to Austria where I had a workshop. Bonny had read some of the books while working in the library, and knew that it would be an energy-consuming five days. But maybe it would be her only, and last, chance to meet some people who obviously were not afraid of AIDS patients, and who knows, she may find someone who would visit her one day when she was totally bedridden and needed more help.

Bonny arrived a few minutes after we started our workshop. A hundred people, of all ages and backgrounds, were already assembled in one big room. Most were very tense and nervous. Some were in wheelchairs, some on improvised stretchers, others sat on pillows or in chairs. I informed the group that this was "their week," their chance to become very honest with themselves. They were not to play therapist with each other, even those who were by profession therapists; they only had to pay attention to their own reaction of what they were going to witness. "As a special bonus," I mentioned, they would "have a chance to spend those days with an AIDS patient." If they had any fears, that would give them an opportunity to face them, to deal with them, and hopefully leave on Friday with a different attitude about those patients. One hundred pairs of eyes looked around the room to "find" the gay man who might be the AIDS patient. Nobody was sure which one he was. No one suspected a young, pretty woman, who hid behind the group, leaning weakly on the wall, her eyes filling up with tears. She had never heard anyone refer to an AIDS patient, as a "blessing." A sudden sense of hope came up in her; maybe she was at the right place.

151

After the formal introduction of the large number of people, she found herself surprised about the openness of so many and the tragedy that so many came to deal with. Many of the women had been abused as children; others confessed to being abusers. Many, many parents were there who had lost or were in the process of losing a child. Some lost a parent or sibling by suicide, some by murder. A young woman was barely able to move—she had M.S. It was a panorama of human suffering and Bonny suddenly felt that she was no longer alone. Even the many doctors and clergy, nurses and social workers who attended shared their private pain and sorrows. It never occurred to her while she was in the hospital that they, too, had private lives, their own private sorrows and nightmares that they had to hide behind a professional front! A great feeling of love and compassion came over her and, for a moment or two, it even occurred to her that this would be a lovely place to make the transition we call death.

After what we call the "physiological break," she knew it would be her turn to introduce herself. She did not know yet what and how much she would share. She remembered that all participants were told not to "rehearse" but to listen to their hearts and allow to come out what needed to come out. She smoked a few quick cigarettes, but was glad when the break was over. And then she heard herself say, in a very calm voice, "I am here because I am dying of AIDS." There was dead silence in the room; you could have heard a pin drop. People looked at her, many with tears in their eyes. Without another word spoken, one of the cancer patients got up from her wheelchair. She was convinced that she would be the first one to leave the workshop. Who would want to share a week in such close proximity with someone who had AIDS? But the cancer patient did not head toward the door. With a staggering, unsure gait, she headed straight toward Bonny. She kneeled down to her and hugged her; the tears intermingled and she found a friend!

It was after the part of the workshop that involves the drawing of a spontaneous picture, which reveals the participant's inner fears and conflicts, that Bonny was ready to share the story of her short life. And she would never forget the moment, shortly after midnight, when the whole group lifted her in their arms and, rocking her, sang "I'll be loving you, always."

A year later, when I was able to talk with her by phone from Switzerland, Bonny told me that she often closes her eyes and hears "our group" sing to her and accept her with unconditional love. She is now, at the time of the writing of these lines, very close to death. She has not been alone since the workshop. Friends, people who had shared this week with her, have visited her and traveled from all over Germany, Austria, and Switzerland to be with her. She has had attendants around the clock. Volunteer AIDS helpers look after her and she even found a sense of humor toward the end. "When I think that my professional colleagues were not allowed to mention my name anymore, I can smile now. Maybe I'll send them all to one of your workshops."

Not one of the one hundred workshop participants had ever been with an AIDS patient, especially a woman, for such a long period of time. We had no problems finding volunteers to share the room with her, and people almost struggled to sit by her during mealtimes. They came from eight different countries and none of them left out of fear of contamination. Bonny knew, at the end of

the week, why I referred to her as "a gift to all the participants," and many of them learned invaluable lessons because they stuck it out and showed great courage and
honesty, especially in view of the fact that this disease was
not very well known in Europe at that time.

Chapter 8

Letting Go

Although this is rapidly changing, the largest group of AIDS patients is still homosexual men. They have carried the stigma of this disease for six years and have buried hundreds of their friends. At the same time, they have educated themselves and have organized extraordinary support systems that now serve as examples to other cities and other countries.

If there is ever a vaccine for AIDS, it will not in the least be the result of their strength and their efforts. For more than half a decade they have been isolated by most communities, have allowed doctors to experiment with them, suffered incredible side effects from experimental drugs, ruined the lives of their families, and participated in anything that promised a cure. In the end, they have succeeded in forcing people to see that AIDS is not just a "gay disease," but affects everyone.

The best known and most successful of the support

systems is in San Francisco. My first patient there was Chuck, forty-two, whom I visited at his house shortly after I saw him on the East Coast:

Q: *You were diagnosed in December? That was prior to the workshop.*

A: Yes, December 7, Pearl Harbor Day. Yes, however, I knew that I had K.S. [Kaposi's sarcoma] long before that. However, my doctor never knew that I had K.S., even though he saw lesions, he didn't recognize them. And even though a dermatologist saw them, he didn't recognize what they were.

Q: *What was the first thing you felt when you were told?*

A: Relief. On December 7, I had a bronchoscopy which determined it, and I received the results of that bronchoscopy right away, within twenty-five or thirty minutes, something like that, that I had a mild case of pneumocystis, and the first thing I felt was "I'm glad," in a way, because it relieved all of that stress that I had been worrying about whether or not I had AIDS. So my first feeling was one of relief, knowing that I had AIDS. The enormity of the situation has been something that I've been trying to deal with since then, but my first feeling was intellectual, and it was relief from the stress and anxiety that I was suffering.

Q: *Did you ever have AIDS panic? I mean, before then, were you afraid that you would get it?*

156

A: The previous April I was hospitalized with shingles, and for a month before I was hospitalized I had sores in my mouth, and I was unsure of my— I had lost all of my self-confidence in my body's ability to defend itself against disease, but I had shingles and it is a malingering illness and so for three months I felt ill. For the rest of the time until diagnosis I never felt really energetic or healthy, and I was very concerned about my health and I was extremely anxious about AIDS and, also, I had a lesion on the side of my head [temple], and I went to the doctor and said, "What is this?" He looked at it and said he really didn't know, and not to worry about it. A while later, I went to a dermatologist as the cyst got larger and he lanced it, not knowing what it was, and he was surprised to see nothing happen—nothing came out. I just ignored it because when he lanced it, the actual size of the lesion decreased a little bit. I just ignored it, thinking it was just some sort of a benign tumor and that's that. On the other hand, I was experiencing fatigue, stress, anxiety over my physical condition so that when I was diagnosed with AIDS—and I might add I had to be very assertive with my doctor. I went to him with a cough I had had for a month, and he said it was bronchitis. Two weeks later I went back to him again and said, "This cough is not subsiding," and it was at that point that he ordered a test, and it was then determined that I had a case of pneumocystis. This doctor treats a lot of people with AIDS. At the time, I believe he had thirty-five patients with AIDS, and yet he didn't recognize the symptoms of pneumocystis that I described very carefully to him, and I had to be assertive, demanding a diagnosis. I got it. I was relieved. Finally, I knew what was wrong, and I was very brave because it didn't really mean my death, although I knew it did, but as I said, the enormity of that is only now hitting me.

Q: *When did you first come to an understanding that you would die?*

A: A realistic understanding that I would die? Only relatively recently. I think I had an actual awareness that I would die because I had AIDS from the moment of diagnosis, but feeling something and philosophizing are two different things, and I never felt that I would die although I could intellectually say, "Well, yes, I am going to die. I have AIDS." And I was very brave. It was only recently that I felt the real fear that comes with facing eternity, whatever that is.

Q: *What are you feeling today?*

A: Today I am feeling anger. I am angry that I'm going to die. Anger is a strong motivator, and I became angry another time and was motivated to start living again, and today I feel the same way. I feel positive and stronger as the result of my anger. So anger is something I feel today. I'm pissed off because I'm going to die, while others aren't.

Q: *When you get angry, what do you usually do about it?*

A: What I have done in the past is that I have cleaned house.

Q: *Do you mean "physically" cleaned house?*

A: I do those things that need to be done. When I become angry— It is a motivator and I do those things that need to be done that I haven't done in the past due to depression, self-pity, or whatever other feelings I may have. So when I get angry, it is generally an anger that I'm going to die and I am pissed off at others because they're going to live, and I feel stronger as a result. The anger, I don't know, produces adrenaline, or whatever it produces, but it does something—I get pissed. I don't want to be dependent on people, and so I do things. I accomplish tasks, which seems pretty reasonable. It's better than going around bashing people, I suppose.

Q: *What worries you most about your present situation?*

A: I think the thing that worries me most is that I will become disfigured and dependent. And that's the thing that I haven't yet come to terms with. Being incontinent, being disfigured—those are frightening situations for me, and yet I understand that they may occur, and I should allow whatever is to occur, to occur. And it's letting go, that's hard. And letting go of anything is hard, especially the most personal parts of you, which, of course, includes your body, and surrendering in point of fact, my ego, and that's very, very difficult.

Q: *That's a big package, isn't it? A big package for all of us. If you were going to give a word of advice to doctors and nurses about the best way that they can help people with* AIDS, *would that word of advice be?*

A: I don't know that I could put it into words, but I think it is terribly important to be honest with the patient. The doctor that I had who diagnosed me with AIDS, eventually, was not honest with me. I had a lesion in my mouth and he never told me. He never recognized, or never told me that he recognized, the lesion on my head. He wasn't honest with me, and he also told me I had about a year to a year and a half to live. I don't think that's honest either because I don't think he knows, and I don't think anyone knows. I believe that a doctor should be very honest and if a patient has AIDS, which is a terminal illness, he should tell the patient that he can only treat the symptoms of the illness and he can do nothing else, and that there is a mortality rate that is 100 percent in five years, or whatever it is. I believe that that is being honest with the patient. Moreover, I believe that among the protocols, and I mentioned this to my new doctor just yesterday, I said that I think immediate prescription of therapeutic massage is essential because it will help the patient deal with stress and anxiety, physical symptoms of stress and anxiety.

Q: *What about family and friends? If you were to give them some advice that would help?*

A: I believe family and friends should be supportive and while it's natural, everyone I suppose, goes through a certain amount of denial. They should understand that AIDS is, in fact, a terminal illness, and not console the person who has AIDS with all sorts of "well maybe there will be a cure, etcetera, etcetera." I'm not saying that one should be totally negative. I think that in a very positive sense, the family should realize that AIDS is a terminal illness and they mustn't wish the patient to get well soon, because it is only denial and what that does is make the patient feel that he can't communicate the reality to the family and friends and that can result in loneliness and even self-hatred. Moreover, I think it is very important that the family understand that it is a virus that is suspected to cause AIDS, and that there should be no guilt label put on the person who is sick because he is sick. Family and friends will feel anger. I have found that people feel anger because I'm ill and they take out the anger in subtle ways on me through either rejection or through not wanting to listen to me talk about death. There's denial, there's anger, there's hostility. We change the subject. We don't discuss reality. We don't discuss situations that will occur. The disease is relentless in its course and I believe that family and friends should understand that and not deny it to the person with AIDS. They should be supportive.

Q: *How do you feel about taking treatments?*

A: Well, I believe that treatments should be— First of all, AIDS cannot be treated. It is symptomatic. Symptoms can be treated and I believe that if there's some impairment to function, palliative measures should be given, but I, personally, don't feel that palliative measures include chemotherapy. If I had a lesion in my throat and had difficulty swallowing, radiation can take care of that. If I had a lesion on the end of my nose that bothered me, radiation can take care of that just as a palliative measure. There's control for pain. There are means of controlling pain. There are means of controlling diarrhea. There are means of controlling all sorts of things, but there is no cure, and no one, at this point, with AIDS will get well, as far as I am told, and so it seems to me that one can cling to hope by having chemotherapy and losing one's hair and having nausea, if that's the type of therapy that is given. To me, I'd rather not spend my time being ill.

Q: *Being well is important to you?*

A: The quality of life is real important and I think that one can die healthy, rather than die sick.

Q: *Depression is a common problem with people with a terminal condition. When you get depressed, or when you get a feeling of being hopeless and helpless, how do you know that you're depressed? And then what helps you pull yourself out of the depression?*

A: I know I'm depressed when my house becomes a mess, when I don't care about things or myself, when I can't concentrate on a task that needs to be done. I respond to the depression when I become aware of depression. It is not a matter of— This is a hard question to answer. How do I know I'm depressed? I think that I know I'm depressed only as it ends. It sneaks up on me, without knowing. Self-pity, anger, hostility, frustration. I get depressed when I don't release emotion. I can't answer that question. It's been difficult for me, for example, to feel in my life. I intellectualize situations and so depression is not new to me, and I know to get out of depression one requires behavior modification. It's a good way to get out, but to become motivated, to change my behavior requires a kick in the ass of some sort and that has to come from within me. Today, I am angry, and I woke up this morning and cleaned my kitchen, which was covered in ants because I had been in a depression for a while.

Q: *So when you have that realization that you're depressed, you're able to give yourself a little boot?*

A: Not necessarily. I may be aware that I'm depressed but I may not be motivated to do anything about it. That's where I need help and that's when I call upon support people to assist me. I am aware that I need behavior modification, and yet to become motivated to modify my behavior is another story entirely. . . . Very often I call upon my priest, you, my friend; others that will help me understand feelings and/or I become angry at myself for not enjoying the days that I have left; sitting around and moping and not doing something will get me angry. There was a time, for example, when I was deeply depressed and I have read somewhere, a couple of places within a few days of each other, I read that the average person diagnosed with AIDS lives approximately nine and a half months. I had, at that time, been diagnosed with AIDS for four and a half months, although, parenthetically, I know that I had AIDS long before I was diagnosed—several months before, in fact. And it made me angry that I was sitting around staring out the window and being depressed with things, and so I cleaned the house, started working in the garden, and started living and enjoying those days that I have left. There is no reason why I can't do many of the things that I did when I was well, except for fatigue or depression, and if depression is the cause, then I only have to get this off of myself—that's the boot in the ass. And then I can start growing again—one day at a time.

Q: *Being alive is nice?*

A: Yes! And while I am alive, I should live, not slowly die. That makes sense.

Q: *Insofar as we are all slowly dying?*

A: Yes.

Q: *Do you pray?*

A: Yes, I do. I have had some spiritual moments and even some religious experiences which scared me because these moments and experiences were very real and very frightening. They occurred during Lent, and during Lent I was identifying with the passion of Christ—more than identifying. I don't want to presume that I was reliving the passion of Christ, but I certainly was empathizing to an extreme degree with death and suffering, and that may have contributed to some extent to the depression that I was in. On the other hand, in a very positive way I realized that I was being shown the way by Jesus. It only occurred to me a few days ago that is exactly what happened. I was receiving images and interpreting them to mean that my time was at hand and I was really frightened and became scattered in terms of trying to do things that day. It seemed like there was so much to do all at once because "my time was at hand," and yet, in fact, my time is limited; I am not going to die tomorrow. I may but I don't expect to, and so I've been given, in effect, in my mind's eye, a reprieve and yet I know that time is limited, and so, I am, realistically, doing those things that need to be done. Religiously and spiritually, I have grown tremendously. Spiritually, particularly. I believe I have always been a spiritual person in my own way, that is to say, I relate deeply to nature, the stars, and the sky, and have contemplated, privately, eternity. As a child, even, I would go off into the woods where we lived and I found a little place where I could be alone and just commune with nature in a very spiritual way, and yet religiously, insofar as organized religion is concerned, I have attended church regularly since diagnosis and it has been revelatory, as well as revolutionary for me. I understand so much more than I did and I find a great deal of strength in the psalms and in the story of Jesus. I have become far deeper spiritually and religiously.

Q: *This helps you to stir up your inner resources and to become more aware of the resources that you have within you to see you through what you're going through?*

A: That's right. I believe that to be true. I call upon religion in a different way than I would have months ago, years ago. Religion actually means something to me now. And I interpret it in my own way, of course, but the devotions that I attend—for example, I go to Evensong each Thursday evening at Grace Cathedral because it is a contemplative time for me, and it is deeply moving. I had a religious and spiritual experience there, in fact, at one time. And I go to church regularly where I learn about things and I can relate to a church calendar. Being a passion of Christ, I identify with it because I am going through my own passion and so, in effect, I am being shown the way.

Q: *Do you ever get afraid?*

A: I have fears and I have felt fear only relatively recently. There is something I've been denying. Fear resides in the solar plexus region and I was talking to my psychologist and he asked me to scan my body and to tell him what I felt. Well, at that point in time, I was feeling very positive and energetic and living one day at a time very well and feeling good, and I was having those religious experiences that were remarkable. I was feeling secure and comfortable and he asked me to scan my body from the tip of my toes to the tip of my nose and I did. I scanned my body and he said, "What do you feel?" I heard myself say, "Fear." I don't know why I said it, but there it was, and he asked me where I felt it, and I pointed and rubbed my solar plexus area and he said that's where fear resides, and I went into a horrible depression after that because I was aware of a new feeling and that feeling was fear. I mentioned that I have always intellectualized situations and here I was having a

166

feeling that I hadn't felt before, or that I had denied myself feeling.

Q: *Are you afraid of dying? Or are you afraid of death?*

A: Oh, I think it is the getting there that's the hard part. I don't want to be dependent.

Q: *We don't always get what we want. We get what we need.*

A: Yes, I'm a little afraid of dying and I'm not afraid of death. I am probably a lot afraid of dying, but I'm not afraid of death. I do believe in a higher level of existence, whatever it may be. Whatever form Eternity takes, I don't know. There is nothing I can do about it, except to accept it, to allow it to occur. That's the hard part.

Q: *So, dying and death, while they're clearly related, are kind of two different experiences?*

A: I would think so. I am experiencing dying right now. I have not experienced death—except little deaths: Disappointments, hurts, moving from one city to the next, years in the past, are little deaths, and that may have prepared me for the big one coming up. I don't know, but in each case there's sadness, grief, anger, depression—little deaths. So I may be more prepared than others because I've moved from city to city, leaving those I loved and familiar surroundings behind, and that's what is occurring now. My house is in disarray because I feel as if I'm moving and so I am preparing for the move.

Q: *And you find that this preparing helps you to take the journey?*

A: I believe that is the case, yes. There is a lot of unfinished business that I have to do and it is causing me to be anxious; for example, I have not written my will. I have not completed the durable Power of Attorney for health care or the Living Will. These are all essential. They need to be done. Now is the time. I've put it off because there is lots of time, and maybe I've really never accepted the fact that I am going to die. And these tasks are *tasks;* they're tedious, and it seemed that there's so much on my mind that it is very difficult for me to concentrate. I need help and you consented to give me help, and my brother-in-law has helped, and I find support wherever I ask for it. But, nonetheless, those tasks that I find difficult have not yet been done. A task is writing a letter to a friend and it is very hard for me to concentrate because I'm preoccupied with all sorts of things. There seems like there's so much to do to prepare for this move that I don't know where to begin. Of course, one must begin at the beginning.

Q: *Finding the beginning is sometimes the rub, isn't it?*

A: Exactly.

Q: *The making of a will, and the Living Will, and Power of Attorney for health care, in terms of all the things that you have to consider in taking this journey, do you find them more difficult to attend to than other things?*

A: No. As I mentioned, even writing a letter is difficult for me because it requires concentration and a steady stream of thought and a beginning and an end. And the will is a very simple task to write out. The durable Power of Attorney for health care is simply filling in blanks and signing my name, and yet those tasks are as difficult, as I said, as writing a letter to a friend. It is simply not concentrated, not directed, and now is the time that these tasks have to be done, and I'm beginning to do them—I'm beginning—and I feel good when I have done those tasks. I don't want to leave unfinished business at hand—when I'm unable to do it.

Q: *That seems reasonable. You are a very reasonable man.*

A: Thank you.

Q: *If you were to die today, what would be your parting words that you would like to say?*

A: Good heavens! I would like to say different things to different people. In general, my message to everybody would be to live, to grow each day, to not be afraid of taking risks and to enjoy life and allow things to occur. In my years, I was so frightened to live, I had so little self-confidence that I was unable to really fully explore my potential as a human being. I believe that while we are alive, we are called upon to live and to grow and to take risks. Without risks, there is no growth. No reward, as they say in the investment business. And also, one has to be true to oneself. In my case, I'm an artist, poet, and a storyteller; a dreamer, a healer; and I became a banker in life because it was expected of me. I allowed myself to be put into situations not consistent with myself, and I feel that I did myself a great disservice. I don't blame myself for it, but my words to everyone would be to live life, not be afraid to grow each day if possible, and to help others do the same.

Q: *What one thing about yourself would you like to be most remembered for?*

A: I would like to be most remembered as being helpful to people. Just helpful.

Q: *What kinds of advice would you give to* AIDS *patients?*

A: Wow! Even though I have AIDS, I don't know that I can give advice to AIDS patients. I believe that AIDS is an incurable disease. The advice I would give those who are suffering with AIDS is to accept that eventuality and to live fully to the extent that they can. I meet lots of people who have AIDS and lots of those people are concerned with which chemical they can take to cure them of their illness, or having crushed grapefruit seed stuffed up their ass, or whatever they think will cure them of AIDS. They're all looking for the great panacea to cure, and there is none. I think that the advice I would give the patient with AIDS is to consider the quality of the life that they have, rather than the quantity of it, since, as you told me, so correctly, we can control the quality, but we cannot control the quantity of life. People with AIDS have a limited life expectancy and that's a big con-

cept to become aware of. I think that one of the
things that I would tell a patient with AIDS, the advice I would give them is to learn as much as they can
about their illness and not delude themselves with
the dream that they're not going to die. For example,
I recall a friend of mine who has K.S. attending a
seminar with me and others on K.S.—he is taking
chemotherapy for the K.S.—and he was shocked and
depressed to find that there was no cure for AIDS. He
has had AIDS longer than I have and he assumed that
by getting rid of the K.S. he was going to get rid of
his immune deficiency and become immune effi-
cient, I suppose, and he was shocked.

Q: *Do you think it is important that* AIDS *patients demand straight answers from their medical providers—the doctors, the nurses, and other people concerned with their medical care?*

A: Yes. I think that's essential, but I also feel that a lot
of AIDS patients don't want to know that. They
won't demand it. They'll say, "Hey, Doc, cure me,"
or they will assume that the doctor is curing them
of their illness. They will simply assume that when
the doctor subscribes whatever— My doctor, I am
fortunate in that the doctor that I now have, is one
who is very straightforward and he offers his
suggestions based on his medical knowledge, but I
have the ability to say yes or no. The doctor I went
to formerly simply prescribed medication and
didn't necessarily tell me why, or what the side
effects might be, or what the end result might be,
any of those things, and if I didn't ask those ques-

tions, he wouldn't give me the answers. He wouldn't volunteer, so there was a conspiracy, in effect, of silence. I didn't know what questions to ask and I'm an intelligent, knowledgeable person, more so, perhaps, than many of those who have AIDS. I know more than they do about medicine and about illness, and if I didn't know the questions to ask, I doubt very seriously that a lot of those other patients will. It is a rare doctor, I think, who understands that the patient must be in control.

Q: *So then, what I hear you saying is that it's really incumbent upon the patient to be in charge of the situation in order for the patient to deal with the situation more constructively and in a more positive healing way, not healing in terms of medication and treatments but inward.*

A: That's right. First of all, I think that it is terrible important that AIDS patients, or any patient, be assertive with their doctor, because doctors don't want to admit failure and the sight of an AIDS patient indicates failure in the eyes of many doctors of their ability to make the world well. I hold a lot of doctors in contempt because of their arrogance in the face of nature, in the face of disease and illness. Other doctors have a more humanitarian approach than those arrogant doctors, and that's the kind of physician I have and I'm really grateful because he's honest. He tells me alternatives and he's very frank.

Q: *And he lets you—*

A: Make decisions. Exactly. Exactly.

Shortly before Chuck died he sent me a tape with his deepest and innermost thoughts:

"Today I'm recovering from an emotional roller coaster. Yesterday was the anniversary of my father's death, and I also externalized a lot of anger and rage and grief with a facilitator known to Elisabeth Kübler-Ross. For two hours I beat apart four West Los Angeles telephone directories with a rubber hose and cried and screamed, heard my voice for the very first time since I was a baby. I was returning to my crib. . . . I was exhausted. And I'm still so emotionally drained from that experience that I don't feel very well physically. I will, for example, cry for no seeming reason or just tears will come. It's grief for me, it's grief and sadness for those I love. It's surrender, me against the ego. These feelings are uncontrollable. . . .

"There's lots of things that go into making or taking a journey or trip. You have to get ready for it. You have to make sure your place is reserved, and you have to get on the train or get on whatever conveyance is appropriate and get there.

"That requires control and that's what's been so frightening to me because I don't know how to get where I'm going, and it's a matter of simply being taken . . . allowing myself to surrender to whatever it is that allows me to get to where I'm going. It's very difficult not knowing where I'm going. It's frightening to me, and it means that I must surrender myself and be content in the knowledge that there is that beautiful eternal part that will never change and never die. It's hard to remember that I have that part in me and that the physical body is nothing more than a shell, a cocoon. That's what I need to remember, to concentrate on the good and the light rather than the dark . . . the trials and tribulations of day-to-day life. . . .

"I'm learning how to live now, ironically, as I die, and what I suppose that means is to give unconditionally . . . to give and not be judgmental . . . to give love. And whatever I give is returned to me. I learn that now in my passion. It escaped me when I was well. I think it's probably because I didn't love myself. I was judgmental or harsh with myself and with others. I didn't experience love. I had been in California for two years or so, and I had written in a journal I kept that my spirit was dead. What did I mean by that? It meant, I suppose, that I was simply not in contact with that essential part of me that is love. I didn't feel loved and I didn't receive love. I was looking for love, as they say, in all the wrong places. And I was depressed and agonizing over the situation in which I found myself, that is to say the low standard of living I had for years. I didn't know what to do. I was ill-equipped for life and that's partially because emotions were bottled up, partially due to other stresses . . . guilt, anxiety . . . all that crap. Not having any friends or an emotional support system. My spirit *was* dead. I lived in a dark, very dreary apartment and that's where I placed myself. I have no doubt that that has contributed to my illness. My own self-destruction was at work. I was destroying myself by not loving myself. I was destroying myself by keeping in anger and not externalizing grief. That evil that was in me, evil in the form of anger that I characterize as evil, negative energy, created the situation that I have to face today. So, in a way, I'm the author of my own destruction. I'm responsible now for living each day as well as I can. I lose sight of that sometimes, and dwell on the self-pity and become mired in depression, suffer physical ills, and

174

as I mentioned earlier, I'm on an emotional roller coaster. So death represents a lot of peace to me, and while I don't look forward to dying because I'm afraid of letting go, I look forward to death, on the other hand, because it represents peace and eternal whatever. . . .

"My most important need, right now, is to communicate. Sometimes words don't really seem effective and I need not to be afraid of today, or at least I need to know that I can make it through the day. Just today. I need rest, peace, and quiet. . . .

"I have been pretty frantic until very recently. I still may be, I don't know. Today, I was able to wake up a little bit later than normal, so I think I got a good night's sleep. At least I felt rested this morning. There are some things that I had mentioned to you earlier, that I want to talk about, and I don't really know how to articulate it, but I know that I am very frightened. Earlier this week I was much more frightened than I am now. I'm worried about K.S., which I've never really seen as a threat before. I have K.S. and I have lesions on my body that are apparent. And I'm getting more of those lesions. I've never really thought of that as a threat. It's because I never really saw anybody with serious K.S. And when I saw a man and he showed me his leg and his leg was all swollen, it really hit me very heavy. That was the beginning of my fear of death. I think of seeing that man and now I really do fear death. . . .

"I have a sense of urgency. I feel that death is near. I felt that death was near around Eastertime, too. It is. That's the thing that is very real. When I say that death is near, I don't know what that means. There is a time, and I have no idea, but I do have a sense of urgency with AIDS. And I also feel a sense of 'not-urgency' to do some things.

I'm willing to not do every luncheon invitation. I have an answering machine so that I don't have to answer the telephone. And I'm asking people now for some help, because I am not capable of doing everything I want to do. . . .

"I've been feeling more removed from my body. When I can relax, I can float. I don't see my body at all now. I have become less attached to my body in a lot of ways. Last night, for example, I was lying down, just relaxing and trying very hard to be out of my body, and trying very hard to achieve that state where I'm not awake and not asleep. A dream. And I became very light and dizzy, almost. And I didn't have a visualization of trees or water, nothing specific like that, more patterns and colors and I was there, lying in my bedroom, but my mind was somewhere else. And then I heard my lover calling my name, Chuck, Chuck. He's in Palm Springs, and I hear him as clearly as if he was in my bedroom. And then I noticed that I was crying. I felt real strange about hearing Danny's voice and I know he was thinking about me, and he's had a hard time being able to go away. He wants to be with me all the time, and I told him not to feel that way, and I think he understands that. . . .

"When I pass from this life I'm going to have a wonderful journey, so I'm excited. I've been excited for years and years about life hereafter, so that has helped me immensely, knowing that my spirit is going to continue to grow, my identity and my spirit is still going to continue to grow, my identity and my spirit is still going to be identified in the hereafter, and a lot of people are hung up in a religious belief. I've made peace with myself a long time ago so that has been another plus for me. . . .

"I want to hit the ground now because it's too terrify-

176

ing being suspended going downhill . . . knowing that I will go down on a daily basis, perhaps. There'll be good days and bad days. Today seems to be a better day than yesterday or the day before. But those bad days are getting worse, and I'm getting really scared. Different physical things may occur. That worries me. They will occur. It's inevitable and I will die, that's inevitable. And I guess coming to terms with that realization, it's terrifying. However, on the good side of things, I've been able to have some ecstatic moments and to really find the common source in all men, and to understand basically where I've been and why I'm here . . . suspended or tumbling into space, crying to myself, and frightened. I know that I was, literally, asking for it, and that my prayers have been answered. And yet I'm not blaming myself for becoming ill, but, on the other hand, I know there's a virus involved and some get sick and some don't and some die sooner than others. I know that. I guess what I'm trying to say is that I don't feel particularly guilty, although there is probably some guilt involved. . . .

"If I die, then I want to be dead. I believe that there are many people saved by Code Blue, but in the case of someone with AIDS, pneumocystis, Kaposi's sarcoma, God knows what other infectious diseases, Code Blue is like—is very similar to what occurred with my grandmother. At eighty-four years of age, filled with cancer, and she had a seizure and a heart attack, and died, and the doctors rushed in with, I suppose, what is called Code Blue and broke all of her ribs in an attempt to resuscitate the eighty-four-year-old lady who was filled with cancer, and who was dead, clinically dead. What a miserable thing to have happen to a body at death. So I do not want to go through anything like that. I do not think it is appropriate under these circumstances for me to be resuscitated, and then keep going for another day, or a week, or whatever, and not get better. At least at this point there is no chance that people can get better with AIDS. There is nothing that I have seen, anyway, to indicate it. I don't want people to think that I have a hopeless viewpoint, but I do have the knowledge and understanding of all the implications at this point and it may sound hopeless to a lot of people. . . .

"My earnest prayer and hope is that I will have been helpful in some way, that my life will be not simply a 'hollow,' as it was. I have had more life and more experiences in the last six months than I've had in my other years, and I have had wonderful experiences and I've done great things, but I've really learned more about myself, more than I ever expected, and I'm able to muddle through all of this stuff, with faith and courage, because there is no other way. And, I guess, I have to have that confidence. As I become more—As I get closer to death, I'm gaining knowledge all the time. I'm learning about me, about my needs, and I hope I'm doing something with myself, with those needs, that I'm just not becoming aware of them and that's that. Although that knowledge is good, it's just like—mind-boggling. And love—I've grown to feel love of me, and others, as I never could have if I did not come down with AIDS. So the terminal illness with AIDS has been my biggest blessing. And it's been a big test. It continues to be a big test every day. . . ."

During my short stay in the Bay Area I also made several hospital calls to see how AIDS patients were taken care of in the different facilities; there were also personal house calls and, finally, at the home of a friend, a number of ambulatory AIDS patients came together, each one sharing what concerned him or her the most. Each patient brought something to eat and we ended up having a lovely picnic, feeling like one big family and celebrating life while we were all able to be together. It was an exhausting day of work but also rejuvenating. It showed me once more how some so-called strangers can assemble, share a common cause, and leave after a short get-together with a feeling of closeness.

One of the AIDS patients, F., was particularly interesting because he compared life with AIDS in New York to life with AIDS in San Francisco:

Q: *You lost a very special person last year, right?*

A: Yes, in March. March of eighty-four.

Q: *What helped you the most during this last year?*

A: I changed environment. My lover and I lived in New York, and twenty other friends died.

Q: *Twenty of them? All within the last two years?*

A: Yes, so I just had to have a change of scenery, and my roommate whom I've known for ten years, since he lived in New York.

Q: *Your roommate here?*

A: No, during the year. But without them I don't think I would have made it. They just gave me an open door to do whatever I wanted, and days when I can't pay rent, they don't care. They're just very special people.

The conversation then went on to children with AIDS *and my dream of starting a hospice for* AIDS *babies.*

A: *I know I only have a short time left and I've been getting teddy bears from people who thought, "If you're sick, they bring you a teddy bear." I would like to donate my teddy bears to that.*

Q: *You also have a cat?*

A: Yes, when my lover died, the cat knew that something was wrong and she would sit on this pillow next to my bed, and she would sit and meow for a while, then she would lie down and cry.

Q: *Yes, cats are often more sensitive than people.*

A: When I went to the emergency room last week . . . she normally gives me a kiss good-bye when I leave, but she wouldn't. She knew something was going on.

Q: *So you brought her from New York to San Francisco?*

A: Yes. Just because all of my friends in New York died. You know what the medical care in New York is like. I'd've been dead by now if I'd stayed there. I went to an outpatient clinic at Saint Vincent's.

Q: *And your friend?*

A: He went there also. He was in the hospital there, too. That's where he died.

Q: *But they don't have an* AIDS *unit. They don't have a special* AIDS *clinic.*

A: I can honestly say, the police—I've seen how they treated patients and I've seen how even medical people refused to take care of AIDS patients. Just taking a verbal history from them, they refuse to do it. They brought me out here to San Francisco to the Shanti houses, which specialize in caring for AIDS cases, because AIDS people in New York had no other support.

Q: *Can you tell me what helped you the most when you were in New York?*

A: What helped me the most? I guess it was my own spiritual values, because I'd lost all of my friends. Twenty of them . . . within a period of two years.

Q: *And that was at a time when New York had no support systems?*

A: Right, and I lost my job because I had to keep calling in sick so often.

Q: *And what did you do?*

A: I was an archivist for the Episcopal diocese of New York.

Q: *And the Episcopal church didn't help you a lot?*

A: No.

Q: *It is very different here. The Episcopal church is one of the biggest supporters.*

A: Yes, I know.

Q: *How long have you known that you have* AIDS?

A: Since August eighty-four. I didn't get an official diagnosis until February 1985 because they wanted to do a lung biopsy and I wouldn't let them do it.

Q: *Good for you. And how did you react to it? Did you know it inside already?*

A: Yes, I could tell, because I had been through all of this with my lover. I was coughing the same way he was.

Q: *And besides your own spirituality, did you have a support group of people who helped you?*

A: I did have a few people at my parish—church—that *seemed* to care a little bit, but it was like when Bob went into the hospital, they wouldn't go visit him.

Q: *So they were afraid also?*

A: Yes. I said, "I'm afraid of this, too. It's not easy for me either to go in there and watch him die, but now is when he needs you the most in his life," and they wouldn't go visit him.

Q: *How long had you known him?*

A: We were together almost eight years.

Q: *So how long after he died did you move out here?*

A: He died in March, and the following January I moved here. I took four vacations though in between to come out here, meet some friends, and see if I

182

thought I'd really like it. And just to get away from New York, and to talk to my roommate, Tom, because we've known each other for so long.

Q: *What's the difference for an* AIDS *patient, not just for vacationing, in being a patient on the East Coast and one on the West Coast?*

A: It's like night and day. New York has nothing. They continually give the answer, whenever you ask for anything, "Well look, we're overworked and understaffed." And I said that "that was an okay excuse at the beginning, but then you do something about it." I couldn't pay my rent, and one of the things they had listed as services was that they would help you pay your rent if you needed it. Well, I would call and they would say, "We don't have any money," so I said, "Do you mind telling me, since you're a public organization, how much your executive director gets paid?" He works twenty hours a week, and gets seventy thousand dollars annually. That's all in donations that people thought they were giving people with AIDS, and that made me furious. I couldn't get any help for Bob. That's one reason why I moved out here, because I knew that there was nothing for me there. No support whatsoever.

Q: *That's beginning to change now.*

A: In New York?

Q: *Yes.*

A: Well, I'm glad to hear that.

Q: *Here, everybody works together on everything, and they really feel like family. Nobody asked, "Are you homosexual? Heterosexual?" Who cares? We're here to help each other and make life more comfortable for each other.*

A: Sure.

Q: *And you find that difference, too?*

A: Yes, they're much friendlier here. You know, we had that candlelight march a few weeks ago. Several of my PWA [Person with AIDS] friends said that they started feeling weak, they wanted to walk it. So they all said that at one point they got very weak, shaky in the knees, and before they knew it, there was a guy on either side, helping . . . and they didn't know these guys, they were complete strangers!

Q: *How many went?*

A: I think there were about twenty thousand or more.

Q: *They came to the candlelight march?*

A: Yes.

Q: *God, is that nice!*

A: It was beautiful to look up and down Market Street. It was just packed with people. It was really nice.

Q: *Yes. See, I believe that most of you chose to have this illness in order to help mankind to raise their consciousness, and to become more aware that we*

184

are all brothers and sisters. And I think if people know that, and that it is going slowly more and more to include women and children, then people begin to know that it is "our" problem, not "their" problem alone.

A: Or like Margaret Heckler said, "We've gotta get this before it hits the heterosexual population."

Q: *It has already hit them.*

A: I know. It's just her whole attitude. It's so sick. She is the secretary of health for President Reagan. Headlines in the *Chicago Tribune* last Sunday were "AIDS Is Not for Gays Alone." Four-page article, but when AIDS came out, it was a byline somewhere.

Q: *Anything you want to share? Anything you want to tell the world?*

A: Well, I guess the only thing I want to talk about is my lover.

Q: *Yes, talk about him.*

A: It's been almost a year and a half now and I still miss him just as much as I ever did. Mark knew us when we were a couple and he knows how much I loved Bob. It never gets better.

Q: *Come to the workshop in August. You can let go of your grief work, okay? If you have no money, you come anyway. You need to come.*

A: I know.

Q: *And you can talk to him and he can hear you. He is totally aware of how you are doing.*

A: Well, I haven't really sort of talked to him, but everybody has his own way of meditating. What I do is I go down into this room where there's a fireplace and two chairs and there's a bright light that's on the other side of the room, which I assume is some sort of divine course, or something. And also he is in that room.

Q: *Tonight, when you go to sleep—I don't know if you pray.*

A: I pray.

Q: *Tonight, when you pray before you go to sleep, ask him to make himself visible in your dreams, and he will come and visit with you. You will see that he is whole and healthy, and dancing, and laughing, and that will probably help you more than any meditation.*

A: This might be a help. It was to me to begin with, but I was at the emergency room last Thursday, at two-thirty in the morning, from severe dehydration. I mean, they were just pumping fluid into me like crazy, and they wouldn't give me any drugs because I told them I had an extremely sharp headache. They said in the emergency room, they can give Tylenol, that's it. So I said, "Don't bother, I know it won't do any good." So pretty soon I must have been hallucinating or something—maybe it wasn't an hallucination. I saw, with my eyes open, or without it, all of

186

these bright colors, and they were colors that I had never seen before. They were just combinations of colors.

Q: *Very beautiful?*

A: Very beautiful. And then, with the colors, people's faces started appearing before me. And then all the colors turned great white and I saw this long tunnel. I sat up and I said, "No, it's not time." I had to shout "No" for quite a while.

Q: *You had an out-of-body experience, but you saw some of the light, some of the colors.*

A: It was incredibly beautiful. It sort of calmed me a little bit about dying because it didn't hurt at all.

Q: *It not only doesn't hurt, it is one of the most beautiful experiences. It's an incredible experience.*

A: But at first I thought it would scare me, but it didn't.

Q: *It's peace and love.*

A: Because then I said my muscles were so tense for so long, and shouting "no," I finally got very tired because I'd been up all night. This was like four o'clock in the morning and so I just sat back to take a nap, and I said, "Okay, do what you want. I can't fight anymore."

Q: *"Thy will, not my will."*

A: Well, whatever, it's just that I couldn't do anything more. I had fought as hard as I could, and I fell asleep and woke up four hours later. So I guess His answer was, "It's not time yet, but I just want to show you a little bit of what you're going to go through so you won't be afraid."

Q: *When it happens again, don't be afraid. Just focus on the light.*

A: I know I'm getting close now because my body is just falling apart like crazy and they can't find anything wrong. The doctors keep doing tests and they don't see anything. Cultures come back negative.

Q: *Do you have a meningitis?*

A: No, I have CMV. There is some neurological involvement and that causes an awful lot of stomach cramps. All of my doctors know I smoke pot and they encourage it.

Q: *We often give it to our cancer patients when having chemotherapy. It really works.*

A: Yes, it really does. I have a friend who has been long diagnosed; he went through chemotherapy. I don't know if there are that many people around who have had AIDS for a long period of time. He's been diagnosed for four years now. He's doing very well. So many wonderful things are happening in my life now. Some of the changes in my life have been really difficult to deal with, like a cane, a walker, and sometimes a wheelchair now, but I really feel, also, that after going through this with over twenty of my friends I know a lot about it, and I really think that part of my job now is to do some educating.

Q: *To teach?*

A: Yes, and I'm going to do that.

Q: *That's what you're doing here; that's part of it. If anything comes to your mind after I'm gone, just write it down.*

After hearing from so many people with AIDS about the lack of response from their churches, it was very encouraging to hear about the help J. received from the Episcopalians:

A: I've been going to the bishop's healing service at Grace Cathedral at the Episcopalian church. It's been very supportive. I go the first Monday of every month to the healing service for people with AIDS. They have the laying on of hands and anointing and it is a powerful moment. It uplifted me and gave me great strength because I didn't feel like a leper once I was in the congregation. The congregation was people with AIDS and people without AIDS who were helping and we all participated.

Q: *One big family.*

A: Exactly; I was part of humanity.

Q: *It's like the candle service you had on Market Street.*

A: Yes.

Q: *That was wonderful. Someone said they had about twenty thousand. And they were all people with AIDS and people who helped support them.*

A: And the church, as well as the small parish that I attend, has meetings on AIDS and healing services each Saturday. I've been attending Evensong, which is simply beautiful music services [held] on Thursday nights at Grace Cathedral and I sit in the choir loft and it's intensely personal, and very simple. One doesn't have to do a lot and there isn't a sermon. It's simply beautiful music and it's been very helpful, very, very helpful.

Q: *One of my patients I saw today had the* Bay Report, *and I think they have a page of all the obituaries of the gay men who died. I think what that* Bay Report *needs is letters from people like you because a patient I just visited is very depressed. All he reads is the obituary of one of his friends. On the other side should be an uplifting letter from an* AIDS *patient to say all of the positive things that happen in the world with them, with* AIDS—*what they learned, how they grew because of it—and not just depressing news. Why don't you write a letter to the* Bay Report *so we can read it next time?*

A: It's a good idea. But there is opportunity. There is opportunity for growth.

Q: *If you're depressed, all you see is the obituary column in that* Bay Report. *If you were to combine that with some positive feedback, you know how that would have helped this last patient. He reads it and he gets more and more depressed and gets like he is giving up. We have two more minutes, then we have to dash. What else do you have to say?*

190

A: I want to tell you that I love you very much.

Q: *Thank you.*

A: And you have been one of the most extraordinary influences in my life and I listen to your tape, "The Santa Barbara Lecture," and I sometimes go to sleep listening to your voice.

C. impressed me the most by his ability to forgive his mother, who, at the time of his impending death, still judged him for his homosexuality. C., on the other hand, had learned that carrying a grudge is a waste of energy and struggled through many issues of his childhood. Ultimately, he was able to forgive his offenders and, within a very short period of time, love unconditionally:

A: We really don't die, it's just a sloughing off of this body.

Q: *A transformation to a much better life.*

A: Yes, we're just moving on to another level of life. People in this country aren't willing to accept it as part of life. When you see it, when you really listen to those words as part of life, in other words, "it's all life," nothing but life, it's all spirit.

Q: *We just shed the physical body when the time comes.*

A: Yes.

Q: *Was it other patients who shared that with you?*

A: Well, a lot of it was just my own energy or intuitive knowledge, but also talking to Shanti volunteers.

Q: *They confirmed it?*

A: Yes.

Q: *How is your family coping with it?*

A: Well, that's part of the wonderful thing, too. I had shut myself off from my mother during the Briggs Initiative, when I found out how she voted, and I just said, "I can't associate with this kind of person anymore." But, again, what really came through to me, through all of this . . . going to the other side is just so remarkable that to me the important thing is forgiveness.

Q: *That's right, and to love unconditionally!*

A: Right.

Q: *No matter how they vote.*

A: I called my mother. . . . I finally just decided because I think this is really important, too, she is still my mother . . . like when I called her that Wednesday night before I was discharged from [San Francisco] General this last time, she said that she still thinks it's bad and wrong to be gay and so on, but *now* I can accept her because, over the years, I have come to accept myself and now I know, I know that I'm not a bad person and that there is nothing wrong with me and I'm not sick or perverted or corrupt or whatever, and because I can accept and love myself then, even though she doesn't accept me, I can accept her not accepting me.

Q: *So you have come a long way.*

A: Yes.

Q: *Who helps you most right now?*

A: Well, my friend. He's been a great help to me.

Q: *How did he react to the diagnosis?*

A: Well, he's been pretty level-headed about it. In fact, I'm wondering . . . I think the other night when we were together, he came over and gave me a massage and I don't know if I really like his having asked me if I would—but again it's sort of an affirmation of my dying—he said I hope you will communicate with me after.

Q: *After you die? Do you feel he's too glib about it?*

A: Perhaps, but he's been a great help to me. He was a great help to me in communicating with this lawyer who, again, voluntarily helped me through my bankruptcy. I was in the hospital and he served as a messenger.

Q: *You went through bankruptcy while you were in the hospital or what?*

A: Well, I put the papers together during the three months I was home sick and I filed before the diagnosis, but then I knew from the timing, when I got in the hospital I told J., I don't know what I'm going to do because the hearing—When I first went into the hospital, I didn't know when the meeting of creditors would be, but I was afraid it would be while I was in the hospital and then I would have to communicate to the court and I didn't know how to do this stuff and so it was like, one of the blessings was like out of the blue. J. meets this lawyer who's willing to do all this stuff. He wrote a letter and put together all these papers to be signed, requesting that I be—because of my sickness—I be excused from the hearings. And then the lawyer asked J. to see the original papers that I filed to—

Q: *And he finished the whole bankruptcy stuff for you?*

A: Yes.

Q: *You see, we call that "divine manipulation," not co-incidence. You always get what you need at the right time.*

A: You see, J. has been so helpful to me all through this. Watering the garden; he cleaned my apartment while I was in the hospital. The important thing is I think the spiritual awareness . . . it's just good not to be afraid.

D. was the most active member of our group and the oldest and longest survivor. He had gone through almost everything an AIDS patient can go through (medically speaking) and had received one diagnosis after another. Both verbal and high spirited, he did not shy away from sticking his neck out to help his fellow man when he

194

*discovered some gross injustices. An activist and sup-
porter of many a patient, he mobilized all sorts of resources to get what he regarded as fair treatment—not
only for himself but for others. An overnight experience
in the city jail showed him how dreadfully and utterly
dehumanizingly* AIDS *patients were treated there. This
led to his visiting the mayor of San Francisco and ultimately suing the city.*

A: I'm D. It all started in 1983 when I had an attack, a
violent attack. It put me in bed for three days and I
went to the hospital, and by the third day I had the
symptoms of hepatitis and I told them I have had
hepatitis before. They said, "Well, the only other
thing it could be was gallstones. But you are a white
homosexual male, it's hepatitis!" And that's the way
the doctors write it off. Anything that looks like hepatitis, if you're a homosexual male, that's what it is.
"Go home, drink a lot of fruit juices, rest, and come
back in six weeks and we will do another blood test."

Q: *What was your attack—you said you had an attack—
of pain?*

A: Violent chills and fever. It was there. I kept saying,
"This is not hepatitis. It is not what I've experienced
before." But they couldn't see it; so I came back in
six weeks and the doctor says, "Okay, you look great,
you don't even need to get completely undressed. I'll
listen to your heart—you know, you are very
healthy." So I took my shirt off and he saw this rash
on my back and he said, "Oh, you have some batiki
eye." I asked, "What's a batiki eye?" And he said, "It's

just a rash. Do you have this anywhere else?" I dropped my pants and my legs were covered with it and this had been going on for a year. Well, I was arrested two weeks ago, and when I was arrested, they asked if I had any medical problems and I told them, "You know, I have a seizure problem caused by my diagnosis and my medication." I also just had a viral attack earlier so I was on a course of prednisone and in the morning the judge dropped all the charges and then I was kept for twelve hours and put in a cell and verbally abused by the police. They were going to keep me another twenty-four hours and I was denied medication and while I was there, the other prisoners were going, "He's sick," "Oh, don't go near that one, he's sick." Well, I've been around a lot of sick people and that didn't bother me and so I went up to talk to these people and some of them had been sitting or lying there for six days, not getting medical treatment.

Q: *Where was that?*

A: This was in the San Francisco City Jail.

Q: *Why did they arrest you in the first place?*

A: Because a friend that I was with insulted a policeman and I was fine. I was with him and then this policeman moved forward and very provocatively, on purpose, moved forward because I said, "Let's get out of here, let's resolve this. I have a medical problem and I want to get to my medication." And this policeman moved forward and very deliberately said, "Well, I think Jerry Falwell is right, all you homosexuals need

196

to die as soon as possible" and then I insulted the policeman and was taken to jail for a misdemeanor and booked, which I have never had happen before and to make a long story short: After a judge drops all charges, you're supposed to be out of there immediately and that's when they sent me back to that cell and another cell and it's all being investigated now that because of AIDS I was being persecuted. My point is that I saw people certainly more sick than myself in there and that's why I'm pursuing it.

Q: *And without medication?*

A: And without medication. I was being denied a nurse. I was supposed to be medicated. The prisoners, you know, were afraid of these people because they were sick and they were saying, don't go see them. I went over and talked to these people. Some of them had very serious illnesses. One with AIDS, I know, and one might have had leukemia or something. What was interesting was that they were medicating other prisoners for insignificant things and they picked out other prisoners that they were afraid of and stayed away. So when I got out, I went straight to the mayor's office and I said, "I'm a citizen here and I have a right to talk to you. I need a guarantee that this will no longer happen to straight or gay prisoners." Sexuality is not the issue, it was just that I saw it in this particular gay cell that they have which is also the filthiest cell that I saw, and it's just general abuse. You see this is what I am working on now.

Q: *So they had a special cell for gay people?*

A: Yes. I think they do that partly so that gays don't get harassed when they are mixed in with other prisoners. They ask you when you're put in jail if you are gay or not and if you say yes, I think it's partly for your protection.

Q: *Has this happened before* AIDS?

A: Yes. It's been called a queen's tank, and the queen's tank is not nearly what one would expect. Well, what was interesting was when I was taken to court, I looked into the other cells and they were immaculate, but that cell, I wouldn't go to the bathroom in. Thank God they didn't hold me longer, because what was frightening to me was that I should never have said that I had a medical condition and I wouldn't have received this treatment.

Q: *And you also wouldn't have seen what happened. You know this happens not by coincidence, this happens to make some waves.*

A: We have an ethical problem here, and I said if you will guarantee to me that this medical mistreatment will not occur, with a public apology, I will not bring the city to suit. But I can't live with myself if I don't have a guarantee that what I saw is going to be eradicated. Well, now what's happened is that I received a letter from the mayor saying, "I think we'll make this public," so they are going to carry it a bit farther than I would have, but I said, "I can't live with myself without knowing if this treatment stopped. It's wrong and what I saw was wrong and it needs to stop, and I'm not concerned about suing for money," though I did tell them I wanted $5.85 for the bus fares that I needed.

Q: *That's a modest compensation.*

A: And I may stick with that.

Q: *Two-fifty an hour?*

A: Minimum wage.... There's a principle involved, not money . . . there's a principle involved. It's in the most recent *Sentinel,* on the front page if you want to read what happened. But it was a new thing for me: medical abuse. Getting a life-threatening diagnosis and being abused. When I got my diagnosis, that was shocking, but you're also shocked when you get arrested.

Q: *Have you ever been arrested before?*

A: Once, but it wasn't serious—no big deal—and this time I was abused and told to die, and it hits you. I was arrested four years ago for bringing a beer bottle from the High Beam down to the street and I was obviously gay. They handcuffed me and put a billy club over my genitals and lifted up underneath my crotch and walked me down the street like that. And I wrote to Mayor Feinstein and five supervisors and the Harvey Milk Club and to the police commissioner because I felt like I wasn't doing anything. I wasn't belligerent; I was standing my ground. I felt like somebody's going to say, "Get up against the wall," you know such and such and I'm going to say, "Wait, now what did I do?" And they saw that as resistance because I was gay. They marched me down the street like that and took me to jail. Luckily, between the place where they picked me up and the jail, I said I was a child-care worker and I said, "Look, I don't have hostile vibes, and I don't know why you're doing this. I work with kids and I think you're making a terrible mistake." By the time they got me down to the jail to the holding tank, they let me go. I mean I was in there and out of there in five minutes. There were five friends with me and they came down to pick me up. I really pushed it because I feel that this goes on all the time, and I have a young friend who's a black gay, and it is like ten times worse because he's black . . . well, "I don't think you make any money . . . and did you pay taxes last year?" It's like extreme harassment.

R. brought up an important issue with which many homosexual couples have to deal, namely, the inability to count on any financial security when one of the partners dies of AIDS. R. had shared his life for many years with one partner and has always supported him. Being a federal employee, he felt comfortable to live on his reduced premature retirement funds, but worried about his partner who was ineligible for financial support.

A: My name is R. I was out at a conference in Leesburg, Virginia, the week of April 30, and I noticed I was very tired and my appetite went away on Thursday night, but I explained that away by saying that there was jet lag and I was in an institution and institutional food is always not very good. Then I stopped in Chi-

200

cago on Friday night to see a friend. I had trouble
waking up to go to dinner and a little buzzer went
off in my mind that something was the matter. I
came back to San Francisco and went to the doctor
for a prearranged physical on May 7, and on the
evening of May 7 my breathing changed. So I
thought something was seriously the matter, but I
did something that I'm ashamed of right now. I told
my mother I was going to go out Thursday night and
had sort of a last fling because I thought things were,
perhaps, not right. Then on this past Sunday, we
were out shopping at the video store and all of a
sudden I felt like I was going to pass out, so I went
outside and sat down under a tree and when I felt
well enough I called a cab and went home. So [on]
Monday I called the doctor and the doctor told me
that my liver tests showed an elevated liver enzyme
count, and that he thought maybe I had chronic hepatitis and he wanted to see me again in three weeks.
Well, one of the things that was going on was that I
was having a lot of trouble staying warm. I was shivering all the time. And my appetite was gone. My
mother even commented on that, being very worried about my appetite. The idea that it was chronic
hepatitis went a long way toward resolving all of that
fear that I was having. I stayed home from work that
Tuesday and Wednesday because I was shivering so
bad at breakfast, and on Wednesday I got up and took
a shower and after the shower I was just exhausted
and having a pain in my lower right side; all these
things would have been explained by a diagnosis of
hepatitis—the shivering, the pain in the lower right
side, everything except the breathing. Well, I called

the doctor again on Wednesday and said, "Look, something just isn't right." I didn't get the doctor, I got the medical technician, and he said, "Well, it sounds like a flu that's going around." So I stayed calm again until Friday night when we went to the symphony, and climbing the staircase to the symphony hall just about did me in. And on Saturday morning I got up to feed the cats and I opened a can of cat food and as I got a whiff of the odor from the cat food, I passed out on the kitchen floor. I got an appointment for two o'clock on Monday afternoon and I had a list of ten symptoms, including the loss of breathing power, that I couldn't take a deep breath to even blow my nose. The first thing the doctor asked me was when did the breathing change. And right there and then it was like, "Oh shit, this can't be happening," and it was two-thirty in the afternoon and he sent me for a chest X ray, and as I was walking over to the chest X ray I saw that he had written down pneumonitis, so as soon as I got back into his office he walked into the examining room and he said, "You have pneumonia," and I said, "Is it pneumocystis?" That was four-ten in the afternoon and my lover gets off work at four-thirty and has a thirty-five-minute commute from Menlo Park. I thought about giving him a call right away but then I thought maybe I would be better off to wait until he got home.

Q: *To tell him personally?*

A: Yes, although I didn't do a very good job of that either. I mean, he walked in and I said, "I've got bad

news and you'd better sit down," and—like a fool—
he stayed standing. When I got home about ten to
five, I called two of my friends because I was just
falling apart. So we went into the hospital the next
day, and on Monday I could walk up- and downhill,
but on Tuesday I couldn't walk downhill. My breathing had gotten like it was when I checked in the
hospital. I was gasping for breath. So they did a bronchoscopy, and then about eleven the next morning
the doctor came into my room and this doctor that
I have is very direct.

Q: *Was he nice, and a person you trust?*

A: I feel very comfortable with him because he is very
direct, which I appreciate. I got to thinking, you
know, he's got his problems telling people that they
got "it." Anyway, he came in and the first words out
of his mouth were, "Well, the diagnosis of pneumocystis— The bronchoscopy was positive." My lover
broke out into a cold sweat and started crying and it
was all I could do to turn over in the hospital bed. It
was like, "Okay, that explains these things."

Q: *And how have you been doing since then?*

A: Well, I was on Bactrim, and I felt kind of cheated
because after six days on an IV they put me on an oral
dose and sent me home. And I had asked the doctor,
"What am I going to do at home, sleep?" And he said,
"No, you can do whatever you want." Well, I felt
kind of cheated because, in fact, I felt very guilty. My
parents drove down from Seattle to take care of me
when I came out of the hospital and I thought I was

going to have energy to sit and talk with them, and that we could talk about things like my estate and what to do, and it was all I could do to get up and go to the table and eat and hope that it stayed down and go back to bed. . . . I just had no energy. People would call up on the telephone, people I have talked to since I've been off the Bactrim and feeling better, and they would say, "Did you know that was me on the telephone?" I kept a book by the bed so that I'd know who called because I really said, "Hello," "I'm doing fine," "I have pneumonia," "I can't talk," "I can't keep awake," "I gotta hang up," "Good-bye." You know, I just have no energy. Since that time, last week, I was very depressed, I have a lot of fear. May 20 was the day I went to the doctor, and thank God for the support groups.

Q: *When do you have the support groups?*

A: My lover goes to the Shanti support group on Thursday nights. After his initial devastation, he was really very supportive. It is unfortunate the day that he called—almost everybody's been supportive except his father—he called his father to tell him that I was sick and his father's reaction was "Get out of there quick, get out of there right now." And that's been sort of hard to deal with, the desertion of the family.

Q: *Did K. help you to get over the first shock?*

A: Well, K.'s into a support group and just listening to the other two couples in the support group really helped to get me outside of myself. I was beginning to get trapped inside of my own mind. Last week I felt like I was sitting around, waiting to die, waiting for something else to happen. This week I have been much better. I have gone to my employers and they have agreed to let me come back to work.

Q: *What kind of work do you do?*

A: I'm a bank examiner for the comptroller of the currency of the U.S. Treasury Department.

Q: *That was nice that they let you come back to work.*

A: Yes, but my job requires real high energy, ten-hour days, super-high energy, and I can't go back to the job that I was doing because I don't have that kind of energy now.

Q: *So what did you do about it?*

A: They're going to try to find an office job for me.

Q: *Which is less energy-consuming?*

A: Yes. I've been with the government twelve years, and the first day that I was in the hospital, the lady that I called when I got home from the doctor, and had the diagnosis, I had her check into disability retirement right away. It works out that I can retire at 40 percent of my salary, and I'll be able to keep my life insurance benefits and I think I'll be able to keep my health insurance benefits.

Q: *So you're one of the lucky ones?*

A: It's like having a career paid off. Mostly I worried about money all my life; my dad was a salaried employee, middle-upper manager, and that's what I am, so I was starting to plan for when I was going to retire. I was starting to save money.

Q: *Now you don't have to save money.*

A: That's why I wrote that down on your questionnaire. Now I no longer worry about being fifty-five. I still worry about money. I worry very much about what will happen to my lover if I die, and he doesn't have my income to support him.

Q: *He will get help. He will get what he needs.*

A: Except that it has been a lot of worry, because for seven years I've taken care of him.

Q: *That will help him to grow and become more independent.*

A: I never used to pray too much, but I sure find that I go to bed at night and I end up praying for twenty minutes. And I pray to God that my friend doesn't get it because he doesn't have all the insurance. I mean, we would be "up the creek" if he got sick. We would have to declare bankruptcy right away.

Q: *There are financial programs that will help you out.*

A: My Shanti counselor just told me the other day he thought that we could qualify for Medi-Cal and still keep the house, but it's been a concern. I've been concerned about whether we should just sell the house and get the hell out from under those obligations.

Q: *SSI—Social Security Insurance—will help you if you have a life-threatening illness. SCI is the California state disability, and Medi-Cal is the medical assistance. They can give you all the information you need. They'll bring the counselors into the AIDS Foundation so you don't have to wait in line at the Social Security office.*

A: Well, see, I am not eligible; neither is my lover because we are both federal employees. I am covered under the federal guidelines, but my lover has only worked for them for two years and you need to work there for five years to qualify for disability retirement. What they would do is put him on leave without pay so he could keep his medical insurance. He would have to pay the cost of that and there would be no income coming in. I make enough money, so as long as I'm working at full capacity I can afford to support both of us if I need to. We may have to sell the house and the car.

Q: *When two males live together, you don't get a pension plan like a widow would get with a husband?*

A: No.

Q: *They've not gotten to that yet? If you have lived together for a certain number of years?*

A: No. They've done test cases in California trying to arrange for that. And in San Francisco—if one of the lovers dies, even if they've been together for fifteen years. Harvey Milk was shot. They took it to court. I believe that his lover couldn't get anything. I think

207

that with the teacher retirement system, you could.
. . . Something that I think happens—you know, I've
been diagnosed for a couple of years—is that your
life-style will change and it can be fun. I know that
sounds strange. It's a challenge, learning how to live
on a different income. You learn to appreciate different things, and you can either see it as "Oh, I've lost
everything" or "Wait a minute, maybe I can only
afford one flower instead of a big bouquet." It's a
challenge and I think that what I've seen through the
couple of years that I have seen a lot of patients is that
you can regret it, or you can almost—it becomes almost like fun. I suddenly know what a flower looks
like. I never did before. . . . When I went to see my
boss yesterday to see if they had worked out an ac-
commodation, when I told him what the problem
was, he said, "This is terrible news," and then he said,
"If I were in your position, I would quit my job and
go and do the things I wanted to do." But, as I said
to K. last week, I'm just now beginning to cope with
things, and like last week I didn't even want to leave
my house. My house represented safety, and now I
want structure back in my life because now I sleep
until ten o'clock and I can't think of a reason to get
up so I pull the sheet back up over my head and bury
myself "in the sand" for a while. I don't feel guilty;
I don't have a guilt trip anymore. I am ill. I love
myself very much. I have to take care of myself. If I
want to sleep in until one o'clock, I give myself 100
percent permission to do that and I don't feel guilty
about it. I feel like that's one of the most negative
things you can do, really. Accept that you're sick and
you have to treat yourself like you love yourself so
much, you let yourself do anything.

Q: *King for the day. Any negative thoughts—fear, guilt, shame—ruins your health. You have to remember that. If you want to get rid of any negativity, come to one of our five-day workshops, as long as you have the physical energy to do that.*

A: Something happened after I got out of the hospital [when] I went to the place where I worked just to visit. I know my life has changed now and it is very interesting, of course. This was early after my diagnosis. I watched them wash all of the pencils I touched, and where I was sitting, and I knew that when I walked out of there, they'd throw all of those things away. They probably took a Kleenex and cleaned them off.

Dear Edward,

Since my last visit with you at the hospital, I have felt a strong need to write a long letter to you about some of the many things we have talked about.

Above all, I must tell you how moved I am by your suffering, and I want to be sure you know how profound my admiration is for the way you are handling your battle with AIDS.

I am filled with wonder by your determination to persevere with appropriate treatment. Although you have repeatedly faced the enormity of your problem, you continue to explore every possible avenue of remission, whether it is a macrobiotic diet or vitamins or chemotherapy or psychological conditioning or spiritual power or experimental medication.

You frequently telephone your friends to stay in touch with the world you know best and to claim their support. You refuse to cop out and pretend that the world has passed you by. You reach for any food that can help you to gain back some weight. You try to exercise each day, even if it is only for five or ten minutes. I see all this and I am awed by your courage.

You also have my unqualified respect for the way you have faced up to the issue of how you contracted this disease. I felt like someone had hit me in the pit of my stomach when you told me you were reasonably certain about how you got it. You blamed yourself for not being more intelligent about your sexual behavior at the time. You knew about the danger of AIDS, but it was not as prevalent then as it is now, and the consequences were not as lethally clear.

I have seldom known anyone who is as balanced as you are about the cause of a life-threatening illness, especially when that cause can be traced to another person. You tell me you were just as responsible as the other party, and that there is no point in wallowing any more in guilt and blame. You often say, "Let's get on with the treatment." How long did you wallow, Edward? We weren't in touch at that early period of the illness. I shudder to think what you must have gone through on that issue. You are marvelous in the way you claim all the help you can get. I wasn't in the least surprised when you told me what you said at your last session of the Sloan-Kettering group. Instead of allowing the period to be overwhelmed by the imminence of death, you fought back. You hoisted a banner of battle. "Fight the disease," you pleaded. "There is help out there. I've [tried] acupuncture. It relieves some of my symptoms. I am about to join a spiritual healing group; I know it will make a difference. If you aren't happy about the quality of medical attention you are getting, do something about it. I'm lucky. I have one of the most supportive and caring physicians in the city. There are a lot of great people around us, sharing our plight. Find one of them. If you aren't getting the kind of love and understanding from your family you wish you had, change it or accept it. There's plenty of kindness and love right in this group if you ask for it. Again, I'm lucky. My family is great. They are generous and loving. I haven't felt rejected by one of them, and I have two very special friends who spend loads of time with me when I need them, day and night. I think the key to my good luck is that I don't mind asking for good things."

I can hear you saying every one of those words. They come from an Edward I know and love. Yet, you and I know there is another Edward, the Edward who can be drawn toward the black hole of final despair when the disease throws you into the hospital, gasping for a single breath, as it did only a few weeks ago. Nonetheless, only eight days later you were listening to tapes of positive meditation and faith!

I am overcome when I think of your journey, Edward. We both know that however brave your battle against the disease is, it is still one of the most severe forms of anguish anyone can experience. First, there was your awareness that you are different sexually from anyone else in your family and from anyone with whom you grew up. Those years before you declared your sexual identity as an irreversible fact must have been years of intense loneliness and unspeakable confusion. We all yearn to belong, but your belonging was under the judgment of the majority. At the beginning you can only have felt surrounded by an icy circle of isolation. Thank God for the peace you fought for within yourself as time went by, and thank God for the wide circle of friends in which you have moved for the past ten years.

> **None of us is so unique as to be exempt from the human condition.**

Having AIDS now must be a repeat of those early years. Once more you are afflicted with a stigma that sets you apart; only this time the stigma carries with it the dreadful burden of our society's panic and phobia about the disease. You are not only not accepted for your sexual orientation, but you are feared as a carrier of death! Yet, you manage to maintain a consistent attitude of compassion and understanding! I recall being with you when you were buying some necessities at a grocery store. Your appearance fits the image so many of us have of the AIDS-afflicted patient; people suspect your condition at first glance. You simply ingnored all those looks of hostility as we moved through the grocery store, babbling away to me about a play you had seen recently on Broadway. How have you escaped the debilitating effects of feeling victimized, Edward? I have seen you angry and repulsed by the attitudes of the public, but it never lasts. You often say, "I can't afford to waste energy on being angry about the public outcry."

However, Edward, what I really want to write about has to do with the two deepest relationships of your life. I am thinking about your relationship to your mother and your relation to your soul.

You have been superb in your effort of affirming all the positives you could find in your life, and in a general face-saving way you have also handled your relation to your mother with such grace, in spite of many scratchy incidents along the way these tough two years. Underneath your style of courtesy, however, I have sensed a deep need in you to have your mother's love and approval, and I have felt your anger over the absence of that support in the way that you desire it. I feel your anger is like a lion in chains. Edward, you can't help what you feel. Don't apologize for your feelings, but let's get them on the table with your mother! All of us aim our fire against those who are dearest to us when we are hurting badly.

> **The journey of the soul is everlastingly determined by our choices. It begins with us and it ends with us.**

It is clear to me that the most conflictual aspect of your life is your love for your mother. I have talked with her at length about your condition, as you well know. Most of your life in the past twelve years has been led apart from her. I doubt if she knows even 5 percent of your experience in that time. I'm sure you know that she made her peace with your sexual orientation long ago. It was not easy for her, nor did it happen without much anguish and excessive self-accusation. Yet, at no time did she reject you or try to inflict a burden of guilt upon you for your sexuality. It was over a year before she came to be comfortable and truly accepting of it after your disclosure. However, some parents of gay progeny never get to that point.

I appeal to you, Edward, to trust me when I tell you that your mother loves you profoundly. Stand on that solid reality. Share your honest feeling with her gently, quietly. Blame is not the name of the game. It ruins everything. Both you and your mother have fought enough inner battles with your nature to know that emotions are prodigiously complex when they are deep as they are between the two of you.

On some of my visits with you, I see your low levels of energy, the constant problems of food and diet, the daily struggle with symptoms of the disease, and yet through it I perceive a long repressed rebellion against your mother coming to the surface. You are asking something from her that she is unable to give. She tells me her response is one of unutterable confusion. She feels the intensity of your need, but she is blocked by something in your spirit from giving you what you want. The result is abysmal distress. She wants to love you and reassure you, but she is overwhelmed by an atmosphere of conflict and barely submerged hostility.

She tells me that no matter what she says, you contradict her. Your experience has made you exceptionally knowledgeable about gourmet food, the theater, dance, cinema, and various luminaries in the entertainment world. Your mother's experience in that milieu is nonexistent. So, naturally, you speak with an authority in those fields that she cannot match. You often treat her as though she were your own age, if not even younger than you are.

> **All of us aim our fire against those who are dearest to us when we are hurting badly.**

There is a decision I beg you to make, Edward. The journey of the soul is everlastingly determined by our choices. It begins with us and it ends with us. For your soul's sake, I beseech you to finish this unfinished business with your mother. Find a way to be open and honest with her. Don't give up until the relation is reconciled. Your soul will be mended by that gift. Without it, you will find yourself in a straitjacket of the spirit on the other side, whenever that time comes, unable to move, stuck in a painful isolation of the soul, pleading for the angels of God to release you. Time is radically different in the next world, where we have no choice but to confront the truth about ourselves. Primal relations that are unfinished here have the gravest consequences there.

You may ask what I mean by soul mending. It all revolves around our being. Doing, believing, thinking, feeling, willing, are only facets of our being. As I write about this great mystery, I realize I am writing not only about your soul's pilgrimage but mine as well. It is ever thus. None of us is so unique as to be exempt from the human condition.

One day I went to Amsterdam to visit the Vincent van Gogh Museum. One particular portrait struck me. It was the face of a very old man. His eyes had the look of someone who has seen all there is to see in the cruelty and the violence of human experience. His torn and weathered brown cap sat squarely on his head. His face was lined with creases of infinite sadness. A cry of profound tragedy came from his mouth. The words I heard from him were, "Attention. Pay attention." It was a plea from the other side of the abyss, a voice from the eternal. I stood transfixed by the power and intensity of the portrait. A line of Buddhist wisdom came to me: "Be a lamp unto thyself." The man in the portrait was begging me to be more serious about my destiny. He was telling me that everything hangs upon the seriousness and integrity with which we persevere in the journey of the soul.

I do not know by what grace I have been given three score and almost ten years, but I bend my knees in humble gratitude for that grace. The time that is given to each of us is a mystery. Had I died when I was thirty I would have been so unformed a soul as scarcely to know that I was in the presence of the angels of mercy. Had I died when I was forty, my wounded ego, which I had concealed from everyone, would have held me in its tenacious grip through eternity. Had I died when I was sixty, things done and things left undone, the power of guilt, and the neglect of my soul's destiny would have barred the path of my soul's freedom.

But by the grace of God, I have been given the incomparable gift of time—time to listen, time to be alone, time to bleed and time to heal, time to be silent, and time to wait. With T. S. Eliot, I can at last say to my soul without shame and without fear, "Be still and let the dark come upon you—which shall be the darkness of God."

216

> Time is radically different in the next world,
> where we have no choice but to confront the
> truth about ourselves. Primal relations
> that are unfinished here have the
> gravest consequences there.

To think you have had only three decades to work out your destiny terrifies me, but, dear man, you have the golden gift of knowledge of the end. At thirty, I had no reason to think that the world was not my oyster, but had I seriously thought I might before my next birthday, I would have welcomed into my life anyone who could have helped me to prepare for the next sphere. By thirty, I had dealt with the mystery of death through the tragedy of warfare, as well as in my family.

I knew even then that the sure hope for my soul was through an identification with the boundless, awesome energy that entered the stream of human consciousness was profoundly altered by those "three sad days" from Good Friday to Easter. No teacher, however great, no human being, however gifted, could have achieved that alteration. Only a divine intervention, releasing a God-filled impulse of immeasurable power, could have accomplished that change in the tide of history.

Although I could not have verbalized my experience of Christ in those words when I was thirty, I would have recognized the truth of them, and I would have made it my business to know His will for me in the time I had left on this planet. Each person's time, each lifetime, short or long or in between, is finally none other than this—the crucible in which we shape and reshape, form and re-form the soul we bring back to the source from which we come. There is no greater grace to assist us in that shaping than the Christ impulse that streams into our soul's consciousness when we open ourselves to him.

The pattern of your essential self is woven by the threads of all that you have desired and loved, of all that you have done, believed, thought, felt, and willed since you were born. As long as you breathe, those threads continue to weave and reweave the patterns of the person you are. There is no escape from the process. It goes on whether you recognize it or deny it. Most of the process remains hidden in the depths of the unconscious. At the core of the process there is an essential you that is continuously evolving in response to the impact of daily experience. We, in religion, call that developing essential person the soul.

> **To think you have had only three decades
> to work out your destiny terrifies me.**

Its character, its form, its shape, is our responsibility. It is overwhelmingly the most important task to which we are called in life. I used to think parenthood was the greatest responsibility we ever carry. I know now that, although it is an awesome calling, parenthood is but for a season. Even a parent cannot ultimately be responsible for his child. I have often thought, too, that I was deeply responsible for the people to whom I have given my heart in love. I know now that, although we bear one another's burdens in love, and so fulfill the law of Christ, in the final accounting I cannot be responsible for another person's soul.

I have often wondered what is meant by the text "It is a fearful thing to fall into the hands of the Living God." Now in my later years I think I know. When I pass beyond the gate of death I will fall into the hands of the Living God, and I, only I will be responsible for the core of the person I bring into His fields of praise.

If I have never seriously thought about my inner being, if I have lived always on the surface of things with no attention to the values that sustain our individual and common life, if I have made no effort to understand myself and the pattern of my reactions to people, if I have avoided any insight into the reasons for my behavior and my misbehavior, if I have lived so superficially that I have always been running, running, running away from the harsh problems and realities of primal suffering and social injustice, then I shall know what a fearful thing it is to fall into the hands of the Living God, because I will have nothing to bring him except a thin veil of confused images signifying nothing but wasted opportunities.

> **To refuse to forgive is to reject the other as that person is. As we forgive, so we are forgiven. As we refuse to forgive, so we are unforgiven.**

There is another level I have pondered, Edward, and it revolves around the problem of authority. If I have never accepted any authority greater than myself, if I have regularly put my own will ahead of any other consideration, if I have avoided a commitment to that which deserves my reverence and veneration, if I consistently preferred my own pleasures and fulfillment to any other interest, if I have regarded speech as something to be used for personal gain and recognition regardless of truth, if I have used other people for my own gain and satisfaction with little thought for their rights and privileges, if I have betrayed the trust that others have reposed in me by breaking their confidences or by countless hypocrisies and double-talk, then when I pass the gate of death, I shall know what the fearful thing it is to fall into the hands of the Living God, because I will have nothing to bring him but an empty cup, a chalice he gave me at birth into which I have poured nothing worth saving.

> **I know now that, although it is an awesome calling, parenthood is but for a season. Even a parent cannot ultimately be responsible for his child.**

We become the persons we are by the things to which we belong. If we have never belonged to anything but ourselves, then we have only empty selves to bring to the Living God when the end comes. The nobler, the higher, the greater our commitments, the more and more we become the person God intended us to be. It took me a long time in life to learn in my inward being a truth I heard years and years ago. At last I well know that my being has but one supreme law: I want to belong to Christ as deeply, as utterly as possible, because I know it is only in belonging to Him that I have any hope of becoming the person He made me to be; without Him I have only an empty cup to bring to the Living God.

But we have not yet touched bottom. It is not the

mind, nor the will, but the heart that counts in the end. If I harbor a resentment against anyone if I look back on my life and blame someone else's inadequacy for my deprivations, if I persist in thinking of myself as a victim, a helpless pawn moved about on the complicated chessboard of life's fortuitous circumstances and accidents, manipulated by those who should have known better, betrayed by those I loved and respected, perhaps even rejected by God if I refuse the grace of forgiveness, forgiving and being forgiven, then when I come to the moment of ultimate and inescapable truth, naked and exposed to the full glare of divine reality, I shall find the gates closed.

To refuse to forgive is to reject the other person as that person is. As we forgive, so we are forgiven. As we refuse to forgive, so we are unforgiven. Kierkegaard wrote, "I must have faith that God in forgiving has forgotten what guilt there is—in thinking of God I must think that he has forgotten it, and to learn to dare to forget it myself in forgiveness."

I beg you to dare to forget the barriers of guilt and anger of the past, knowing that if God can forget them, you can too! Don't misunderstand, beloved man, the barriers are better faced before they are forgotten. I am one of those who took an unconscionable length of time to learn that wisdom; but once faced, openly, truly, and worked out as best you can with those who may be involved in the tangle of your life, there comes a moment when you "must have faith that God in forgiving has forgotten," and in that hour of Godlight forgive and forget yourself.

> The pattern of your essential self is woven by the threads of all that you have desired and loved, of all that you have done, believed, thought, felt, and willed.

When I started this letter I had just visited the hospital. I looked at your eyes, glazed with fatigue. I hugged you and kissed your brow. Your head was wet with fevered perspiration. I came down here to my little study near the ocean. I unlocked the door and wept. I wish I could give you more than the comfort of my life, and I guess it is that driving need in me to help you that made me bold enough to write this long, windy letter. I can only add that I believe in miracles, and I believe in that courageous spirit of yours. It may even yet win the day!

As always,

J.

Chapter 9

The Birth of Support Systems

The training of "an army of volunteers" is essential because the number of needy AIDS patients and families of AIDS patients will increase manifold. Our hospitals will not be able to care for of all of them and, besides, they should only be used for active medical treatment, diagnostic workups, and medical emergencies.

According to the December 1986 report from the surgeon general of the United States:

> AIDS is a life-threatening disease and a major public health issue. Its impact on our society is and will continue to be devastating. By the end of 1991, an estimated 270,000 cases of AIDS will have occurred with 179,000 deaths within the decade since the disease was first recognized. In the year 1991, an estimated 145,000 patients with AIDS will need health and supportive services at a total cost of between $8 and $16 billion.

The hospices are in a double bind; many of them are afraid to admit AIDS patients for fear of losing their financial support, which comes, primarily, from cancer patients and their families. Up to now, only 16 percent of all hospices in the United States even accept AIDS patients and few of them are happy about it—except, of course, in those cases where it brings financial gain. It is a sad story but a fact that financial need determines whether or not a facility will join nondiscriminatory hospices.

If it were left to me, I would never license a hospice that discriminated, whether for race, sexual preference, creed, or medical diagnosis.

The other problem the hospices face is that they can only admit patients if they are terminally ill and are expected to die within six months. With cancer patients, this is relatively easy to foresee; with AIDS patients, however, the clinical picture is quite different. They can be deathly ill and on the verge of dying yet recuperate enough in a few weeks to return home. It is an unpredictable disease that can swing back and forth between "close to death" and practically well.

Another issue is the rule that hospice patients must sign a waiver that no active treatment is to be given to them to prolong their lives. This rule was well meant, but written with cancer patients in mind. With AIDS, you can have a very sick, critically ill young person who may rally his strength once more if his acute infection or pneumo-. nia is actively treated. To withhold such treatment would be criminal neglect and not in the best interest of the patient.

Because of these difficulties, I think it is mandatory that we create specific hospices for AIDS patients. As it stands now, they should be brought to a hospice only

224

during the acute phase of their illness, when all medical resources have been depleted. At other times, these patients should be treated and cared for in someone else's home, in their own homes, when possible, or in a group home.

In order to give adequate home care and to staff the group homes we need literally thousands of well-trained volunteers. Years ago I offered such training services to the Centers for Disease Control in Atlanta and have advocated it to the thousands of people who have attended the public lectures I give throughout the world. But little has been done to implement such a project.

I have, therefore, stressed this national (indeed, international) need especially in my workshops, which started seventeen years ago and are well known. I carefully described these workshops in my book, *Working It Through:*

> The workshops began when I realized that, though we were reaching thousands of people every week with the lectures I was presenting, I felt this was not enough. We were not reaching people in a helping way so much as in an informative way. I know the work that had to be done was larger than this. It had to do more with helping people than telling them about the needs of others. But helping them do what? The answer to me was simple, and came from my years of work with dying patients and their families. The answer was contained in every one of my lectures. People needed help, I told my many audiences, in dealing with the "unfinished business." The workshops were developed as a way of offering that help.
>
> Our goal, our purpose, in these five-day sessions is to help our participants get in touch with their

deepest and long-repressed pains, guilt, fears, and shame—and thus their unfinished business. We basically teach them what dying patients usually try to do on their deathbed—and that is to finish their unfinished business so they have no more negativity within them and they can literally live until they die with a sense of peace, serenity, acceptance, and forgiveness for others and themselves.

It became very clear over these last years, working with healthy people as well as terminally ill patients, that our only enemies are guilt, fear, and shame. Such unresolved negativities prevent us from living fully and deplete us of so much energy that even a fight with cancer is a losing battle when we have a sense of punishment, a sense of hopelessness or a feeling of unworthiness to get well. Many of our critically ill patients were able to get in touch with their own self-destructiveness, which had contributed much to the onset of their cancer. They shared their own inner battle or impotent rage, which gradually destroyed them emotionally and physically. They had never felt comfortable enough to share with their fellow human beings who are so often judgmental rather than understanding, who show pity rather than compassion.

In these workshops, more and more of our attendees started to share their innermost agonies—stories of incest, of misuse, of being battered children, of unfairness, unfaithfulness, experiences of mistrust and undue punishment as children. These were taboo issues that they never shared with their fellow man before, and that they carried with them as a heavy burden through life. Their traumas often resulted in a specific choice of a profession in a desperate attempt not only to resolve their own agony and pain but to help others in similar situations.

Many nationally known support systems are now staffed with people who received their first impetus and training from one of our groups. The director of The Lighthouse in England, the first such official support system in that country, started with us, as did the director of nursing at the AIDS unit of San Francisco General Hospital.

That this is the best and most beloved of AIDS units is largely due to the work of David, the assistant director of nursing; Cliff, the clinical nurse specialist; and Allison, the head nurse of the unit.

They have shown great imagination and dedication. They fought for and created the first AIDS unit in this hospital and have been tireless ever since in their care for their patients. They have provided the best support system in the world.

Here is an excerpt from one of my visits with them:

ELISABETH: *David, you are the director of nursing?*

DAVID: I'm the assistant director of nursing and I'm the AIDS coordinator here at San Francisco General. I planned and set up this unit. This unit was created because of nursing. No one was interested in what we were doing here, and it would never have turned out the way that it has if nurses hadn't said, "We want to provide good care to these patients because they're not getting it." And if we had allowed other people to have their way, this unit would never have been set up the way that it is.

ELISABETH: *And now, you see, it makes the whole hospital famous?*

DAVID: I think so. This unit opened on July 29, 1983.

ELISABETH: *You were one of the first people? And you, Cliff?*

CLIFF: Yes, I had been working with AIDS for about a year before. I [am] a clinical nurse specialist, and I had recognized right away that we had lots of problems, the way patients were being treated. I was very fortunate in that there were a number of people here who agreed with me, but no one was willing to really act on it. I then approached the director of nursing and told her that I really wanted to be involved and she said, "I think you're the person to coordinate it; would you like to coordinate AIDS here?" And I said, "Sure." Now at that time they were talking about opening an AIDS unit because they were thinking, "Oh, we have to isolate these people and we have to get them away. We have to protect the other patients, we have to protect the staff, we have to protect ourselves." And I never believed that, even then. I realized, at the time, that we were taking a big gamble, but we were willing to take that, and it's paid off.

ELISABETH: *And the nurses volunteered to work in this unit?*

CLIFF: Yes, I set up specific criteria. I had no difficulty at all in recruiting the staff. We, basically, had almost no attrition rates. None of the nurses ever really resigned. We had one nurse who resigned to go back to art school a few months ago, but even she works per diem, and then we had one nurse that transferred after a year, but, basically, all of the original staff are still here. I think that, in itself, says more than anything.

ELISABETH: *And how many patients have you had here?*

CLIFF: Oh, my God, we have probably had, over the past two years, about six hundred patients on this unit. I think that one day this should be donated to some historical society because of the amazing things that happened here. Relatively, the numbers fluctuate, but we actually have few patients that die here now. Because of what we've done, we are able to facilitate, educate, and create the support. The patients don't want to be in the hospital. If they have to be in the hospital, of course, they want to be here.

ELISABETH: *If they can, they go home to die?*

CLIFF: That's what they want to do, and if we can provide the support, we'll do it.

ELISABETH: *Hi, Allison, I'm glad to meet you. You are the head nurse of the unit?*

ALLISON: Yes. There are so many things that a number of us have wanted to say to you and talk to you about. When I went about setting up this unit, and making the plans for it, I copied daily from your ideas and read your books, and this unit is based upon your teachings.

ELISABETH: *It's unconditional love which is the most important.*

ALLISON: Exactly, and I think that this unit really [exemplifies] that. This is not a depressing place to work. I think anybody who works here will tell you that. You hear laughter here; this is a colorful place.

ELISABETH: *Do you let children and women come here?*

ALLISON: We haven't had any children; we have had women, a couple of them. One was the partner of a bisexual male, and the other was from a transfusion. There's nothing like this unit anywhere. I think that the shame of it is that we have no competition. I think that is almost a disgrace, not that we are in the business for competition, but I think that it would be very healthy and very good if there were other units like this around. I think that it is amazing that, in this area, there's not one.

ELISABETH: *There is a hospice to be completed in January, isn't there?*

ALLISON: Oh, you mean a facility? It will probably not be in January. There's a lot of renovation that has to be done on the building. I'm a member of that parish and everybody's really excited about that. It was controversial at first, but when the congregation voted on it, only twenty-six people were against the idea. I thought that was amazing. Probably about four hundred people voted.

ELISABETH: *Things are changing for the best.*

ALLISON: I can see attitudes changing slowly. They're not changing fast enough. That's part of the problem. I think that people still look at AIDS, and they say it is a gay disease. The most important thing, though, is to get across to them that the way they are going to get it is through sexual contact, that you don't get it from being in contact with regular casual sharing in the same household. Now that we have the antibody test, it is supposed to screen the blood. I think that it was very naive of everyone to think two years ago that it was isolated in the gay population and we don't have to worry about it. We have volunteer nurses. The nurses—they are no different from nurses anywhere.

ELISABETH: *They* are *different. They have no fear.*

ALLISON: They are different because they are very committed professionally. But there are many, many nurses out there that I think feel the same way if we could reach them. More than anything else, I think politics played into it—as much as I dislike politics— in this city, that's exactly why this happened. The gay community is so concentrated and so vocal and involved politically, that's why it happened here and it has not happened anyplace else. The community feels that this unit is theirs and we encourage them. They responded. We are moving sometime next month, probably about the seventeenth of August, to a unit where we will expand by eight more beds.

ELISABETH: *How many do you have now?*

DAVID: We have twelve. We will expand to twenty. We have a consult nurse that sees all of the patients so that they're all tied in with all of the services. Our problem is that we are totally out of space here. We outgrew this unit two months after we moved into it, and where we're moving to will be outgrown very quickly, too. But we are going to feel good for a couple of weeks because we'll feel like we have lots of space. I have traveled and consulted quite a bit. Allison and I met with a whole group of them here just a few months ago. You know what they said to us? They said, "Well, we can't do in New York what you're doing here. There's no way we can do it. What you have here is ideal. It would never happen in New York." And my response to them was, "With that attitude, it never will. You have to make it happen." People come from all over the world to see what we're doing here. It's actually interesting that we had more interest and enthusiasm from people from other countries than we have from Americans. It's amazed me sometimes. I just went to Australia and I was amazed to find how much planning they're doing. I don't necessarily agree with what's going on there, but at least they're planning. The same thing holds true for the major cities in this country, I think you'll be fascinated at the planning that's going on. You may not agree with the things they're doing but at least, and at last, they are doing some planning.

Perhaps my "pride and joy" student is Irene,* who has made quite a name for herself and has received many honors for the outstanding work she did, and still does, with AIDS patients. When Irene attended her first workshop in 1980 she had gone through a decade of great troubles; she had been on drugs and supported her habit through prostitution. It took another three workshops before she could deal with her tremendous lack of self-love, her fears and her shame and her guilt. Slowly there emerged a woman filled with love, and she was eventually able to give to others in extraordinary ways.

In the last five years, Irene has given of herself and

*Irene Smith, now my assistant in San Francisco.

has started countless support systems and trained dozens of other therapists. The last time I spoke with her she was even offering her own workshops. The most recent of her periodic reports speaks for itself:

I would like to share briefly how I came into contact with Dr. Elisabeth Kübler-Ross and her work. After spending fifteen years of my life as a drug user, an alcoholic, and nine years as a prostitute, I found myself so full of pain that I basically had no more room for living. I was advised in 1980 by my mother to attend one of Elisabeth's workshops in Calgary, Canada. It was in this five-day Life, Death, and Transition workshop that I was afforded a safe place to work through a lot of the pain and guilt and anger and negativity that I was holding inside, for myself and for all those surrounding me. I attended three Life, Death, and Transition workshops with Elisabeth in 1980 and 1981, and as I began to clear my own pain, I started to come in contact with the unconditional love and joy and creativity that life is really about. Elisabeth's work has made my life worth living. It has opened me to the love and spirituality that we as human beings are really about, and it has made me want to share that knowledge and that love with others. Wanting to reach out to others, I called the San Francisco Hospice in the beginning of 1982 and began as a massage volunteer.

It was in July of 1982 that I was sent to see my first AIDS patient. I quickly became aware of how the touch therapy not only eased the physical pain and the isolation for Richard, but it also helped to ease the amount of fear that was being felt by his friends and support system. So I requested that the hospital allow me to see the other

233

AIDS patients as they came into the program. In 1983, San Francisco General Hospital opened Unit 5A, a unit designated for AIDS patients only, and in August of 1983, I was accepted as their first volunteer and started going to the unit once a week to offer massage therapy, room to room, to the patients. In November of 1983, I attended the first Elisabeth Kübler-Ross workshop for people with AIDS as a massage volunteer and rendered massage to approximately twenty-four people with AIDS at that workshop. In March of 1984, I went back to Wildwood Ranch to the second workshop for people with AIDS, where I gave massage therapy to approximately twenty people with AIDS.

Each time I came back from one of these workshops, I continued to see the participants on an ongoing basis, doing volunteer massage work. It was in the latter half of 1984 that I went to the San Francisco AIDS Fund and asked if I could please be funded to continue my massage work. In 1984, I started receiving a small amount of funding each month to continue to work with people with AIDS, through hospice, through San Francisco General Hospital, and seeing people in my home and in their homes. I have since begun a training program for other massage therapists wanting to reach out to people with AIDS on a volunteer basis, rendering massage therapy. There are presently twenty-five massage therapists on a volunteer basis with the Hospice of San Francisco. We now have a team of five massage therapists in the unit that has changed from 5A to 5B in San Francisco General Hospital—and one volunteer in Presbyterian Hospital. I am currently offering workshops for people facing life-threatening illnesses, focusing on people with AIDS and ARC conditions.

[As I said, the first AIDS patient I was sent to was]

Richard. I arrived at Richard's home and walked into his bedroom and there was a man who was about five feet eleven inches, who was skin and bones, had big wide eyes, and was crawling across the floor. He said, "Stop, stop, I want you to watch me do this. Watch me, I can make it to the sofa." He crawled from the bed to the sofa, up on the sofa, back down off the sofa, across the floor, and back into the bed. When he got back up into the bed he gave me those great big wide eyes, and said, "Look what I can do; I can crawl from the bed to the sofa," and I knew right then that I wanted to work with Richard.

Richard was recovering from pneumocystis. He had TB, herpes, K.S., thrush infection, and parasites. The parasites were getting to him. He hadn't been able to digest any food for several months and had a severe case of diarrhea, which was the primary reason for his weight loss. That was in July 1982, and I began to do massage work with Richard's legs and feet. As do a lot of AIDS patients, Richard was experiencing a lot of leg and foot pain.

In 1982, the fear level was much higher concerning AIDS patients, and even though there were a few support people around, massaging someone with AIDS, or being that close to them and touching them, was relatively unheard of. So it was quite a wonderful experience to be an example to the support system and the family members that were around Richard at that time—that it was okay to be close. Richard and I had a wonderful relationship. We did a lot of talking. He had an enormous amount of energy and had been a person who had lived with a great passion for life.

He had decided that as he had lived in production, he wanted to die in production, and he insisted on a large group of people around him at all times. Richard talked about growing up, or spending a number of years on Fire Island, and had decided that the life-style that he had led on Fire Island was the main cause of his cancer, or his AIDS. He talked about different sexual experiences that he believed had created the negative space for his AIDS. Richard had been sick for a couple of years before he was diagnosed. I think the most incredible experience, or one of the most incredible experiences, that I have ever had working with someone with AIDS was with Richard during the last seven days he was alive. You know what happens with so many people with AIDS is that you think they are going to die and then they just keep on living.

The heart is so strong and the will to live is so strong that it really does take an extreme level of deterioration before they finally go through the dying process, and Richard actively died for seven days and seven nights. It was my first experience of this type and, therefore, I insisted on sitting right with him for seven days and seven nights, and sleeping periodically on the living room sofa. I believe I left his home only two or three times during the course of the week.

There were three other volunteers there; his mother and father; one healer who did visualization and a type of hypnosis; and a couple of other friends, who would come and go. It was more or less "open house" for seven days and seven nights. It was quite an experience. Richard refused to close his eyes or his mouth.

The first couple of days he was given injections of morphine to help calm him down. He was waving his arms, and talking, and people were saying that the disease had gone to his mind. Being someone who had spent time at workshops with Elisabeth Kübler-Ross, there were a couple of us there who felt that it wasn't so much that the disease had gone to his mind, but that Richard had an enormous amount of stuff to finish before he died, and so we stayed pretty close to him. One of the most remarkable experiences of this seven-day period was when one evening Richard kept drawing up his legs and arms, and people kept coming in the room and putting them down. After everyone had gone to bed, his mother and I sat in the bedroom with Richard and he kept drawing up his arms and legs and, at one point, started talking about it being "very dark in here." So I asked Richard, "Where are you?" He said, "I'm birthing," and I asked, "Are you in the womb?" Richard said, "Yes, I am." I asked him, "What's going on?" He answered, "It's very dark in here and I want out."

Richard assured me that he was birthing and he started talking about things that were going on with his mother at the time that he was being carried, so I felt that it was very important to wake his mother and father up, and that's what I did. They came into the bedroom and sat down and Richard began telling his mother a couple of things that were going on with her at the time he was being carried. One of them (and Richard did have a great sense of humor) was all of a sudden, he blurted out, "Oh, Mother that gas—my God, that gas!" and she started laughing and said, "How did you know?" He said, "Oh, you had the most terrible gas the whole time you carried me and every time you passed gas, it bounced me around!" We all laughed. He gave us an enormous amount of information. At one point, Richard was unable to even hold down water and everyone had gone to bed and once again his lover and I were sitting in the bedroom with him and he basically seemed quite clear and asked for a sip of water to cleanse him even though I knew that he would throw up and that, medically, it was not a good idea.

[But] he asked me [again] to please give him a sip of water . . . and I did. He took a sip and then he asked his lover to give him the bedpan, and he threw up. When he threw up he named a year and an experience, and he said, "That is cancer number one; give me another sip of water," and I gave him one. He got the bedpan, threw up, and he gave an experience, a date, and a name, and then he said, "Cancer number two; I must be clean—I am going to go clean, pass me another sip of water," and this went on for a while. There are a lot of medical no-no's here. He really believed that he was cleansing his body and was going to throw up those experiences before he died. His lover and I simply allowed him to take control of his affairs and be a part of a cleansing that was very important to him.

Richard kept on and on, and his family and his support system became extremely exhausted. I went home for a couple of hours—I believe that was on the fifth day—and when I got back, one of the volunteers took me aside and said, "Irene, I don't want you to be upset but it was thought best that Richard be given an overdose of tranquilizers so that he would not wake up again. Everyone was exhausted and felt like that was the best thing to do." I was horrified. I went into Richard's room and he was lying on the bed uncovered. I sat next to his bed and talked to him and even asked his forgiveness to have been a part of what was going on and that I did not believe it was right, and I have forgotten if it was the middle of the night or the next morning, as it was three years ago.

Richard sat straight up in bed and screamed at the top of his lungs, "I know what you are trying to do, and

238

it won't work." Richard lived and he had a lot to work through, and as we all know, people are going to die how and when they want to die, and when they finish what they need to finish. The next two days Richard was highly sedated and he was trying very hard to talk despite the tranquilizers. I sat very, very close to the bed and he was saying, "Bottle, box, bathroom, kitchen, living room, and light bulbs." The message that I got from him was, "Take the valium out of the bottle," which meant to me, "Do not give me Valium, put me in a wheelchair, turn on the lights, wheel me to the bedroom, bathroom, and kitchen. Let me see if my house is okay so I can die in peace."

He had been bedridden for quite some time and there had been changes in the house since he had been bedridden, and he needed to see his house since the changes, so I relayed that message to his lover. I went home and went to bed. The next morning he was given a wheelchair, and his parents, his lover, and some support people wheeled him around his house so that he could see every room. Then they took him and put him back in bed. He was much more peaceful. The next day, at noon, Richard died peacefully in his room alone, with the support people having gone home and his mother and father in the living room. God bless Richard! He is worth a million textbooks and five hundred years of living.

Richard taught me that patients die when they want to, and how they want to, and they finish exactly what they need to finish before they go and travel on to the next plane. Richard also taught me that patients deserve dignity and control in their death process.

In 1982, when I worked with Richard, there was still an enormous amount of fear connected with AIDS, and patients were experiencing a lot of rejection within the community and the entire society. There were not a lot of volunteers working with people with AIDS at that time, so I decided that I was mostly needed by people with AIDS. Besides, Richard's passion for life, and the struggle to finish exactly what he needed to finish before he died, really excited me! I decided that I could be of best service to people with AIDS so I asked the volunteer coordinator at the hospice if I could go to Unit 5A at San Francisco General, which had opened in the summer of 1983. I asked if I could go to the unit and do massage therapy. They spoke with the staff in 5A and they let me do it. I believe it was in July 1983 when I started massage therapy in the San Francisco General Hospital AIDS Unit, which consisted of twelve beds.

I was one of the first unpaid volunteer staff members at San Francisco General, and to go into that unit at that time with "touch" was an absolute miracle. There was so much fear in the community that even though there were Shanti volunteers that went in and talked with people and occasionally held a hand and did this type of touching, to do full body massage with these people was received like it was a miracle. The love and support that happened, and is still happening, on that unit is also a miracle. It's a real model unit in humanism. The staff works very hard to meet the patients' needs on physical and emotional levels. The one need that is missing is a Screaming Room so that the patient's family and staff alike have a place to deal with their anger and frustration. More healing could be facilitated and there would be less burn-out with the staff if there were a place "to let one's hair down". A Screaming Room is a must and should be considered a basic need just like toilet paper and toothpaste. In the beginning there was a lot of experimentation with patients so far as drug dosage goes with drugs that are being used semisuccessfully now. The treatments were very harsh and I remember one man that literally burned to death from too strong a dose of septra. It was hard in the beginning.

He was literally burned from the inside out, with skin falling off his bones. Some very positive "touch" stories that I remember from Unit 5A: I went in to see my friend, Henry, one night after he had a colostomy. He had a catheter, some chest tubes, and he wasn't doing very well at all. He was very close to dying and I sat down and asked Edward if he would like anything in the way of "touch" and he said he would; he really didn't know how he could move but he would like for me to massage his back. And so I told him not to worry, that I would find a way. I remember lying down beside Henry, taking my arm and very gently slipping it underneath him and beginning to stroke his back slowly, and while I was stroking his back from underneath, I was running my other hand very gently across his chest, after which he really began to relax and soften. A few minutes later, I took my hands and started going very, very slowly and gently down his arm. All of a sudden, Henry looked at me and said, "Ah, this is the way you always want your lover to touch you and he never takes the time; this is the way you always hear that love feels, and you never get to experience it. These are true loving feelings and I'm experiencing them now. True love has no gender, does it, Irene?" God bless Henry! I'll never forget that story.

Another wonderful story about [the unit] was when I went in to see my friend Larry, who was very, very close to death. I was sitting in the staff room and his mother came in and said, "Irene, Larry would like for you to come in and give him a leg and foot massage." I knew that his parents were flying back to Florida that evening and this would be the last time that they would see him so I told her, "Okay, I will be right in as soon as you leave." Well, a few minutes later, the nurse came down the hall, and said, "Irene, Larry would like for you to go in there and give him a leg and foot massage." So I went into the room and said, "Larry, I know that you want a massage and I will be in as soon as your parents leave." Well, Larry took off his oxygen mask and he looked up at me and said, "Irene, you don't understand. I want you to come in here right now and give me a massage so that I will have the energy to visit with my parents this one last time—got it?" I said, "I've got it." I sat down and gave Larry a massage. Shortly thereafter he took off the oxygen mask and said, "Okay, I can do it now; thanks." I said, "You're welcome, good night now." Larry was really beautiful to work with.

So far as the love and support that goes on in the unit, it really is quite extraordinary. There is a regular staff of doctors and nurses, and also a paid Shanti staff. Shanti does empathy counseling. They also do an enormous amount of business that social workers do so far as making people aware of the services and when they are due and helping people arrange for these services. Shanti also has residences for people with AIDS. I believe, at this time, they have six houses. Most of them house an average of four people each. Hospice does the attendant care for these homes. They are very well run and give a very good feeling of home.

In 1983, I also had the good fortune of attending Elisabeth's Life, Death, and Transition workshop for people with AIDS at Russian River. There were thirty-two people with AIDS in attendance. It was quite a remarkable workshop, and after it was over, I had the names, addresses, and phone numbers of thirty-two people with AIDS and I came home and started calling them and setting up massage appointments. All of a sudden, I had thirty-two patients with AIDS!

There was also another workshop. It was a Love and Healing workshop given by the San Francisco AIDS Fund in 1984. There were about fifteen people, plus about twenty-four people with AIDS at that workshop, and I also took those people on. So the latter part of 1983 and all of 1984 was extremely busy for me. I was seeing as many as fifty people with AIDS for massage therapy. During the year 1984, until this part of 1985, I have been through seventy-four deaths with friends of mine due to the condition of AIDS.

One of those deaths that I would like to tell you about, which was quite an incredible experience, was with my friend Tom. Tom's lover, Bill, was his sole care person at the time that we met at the Russian River workshop. Bill took incredible care of Tom, who was recovering from pneumocystis and not doing well at all. The doctors actually thought that he was going to die much sooner than he did, so he was put on a very high dose of morphine for the pain. But Tom continued to live, and even though the doses of morphine got extremely high, they did not help his pain. I would see Tom twice a week and do reflexology. Tom was a man of Hindu soul and it was really part of the Indian culture, as far as his religious beliefs went; a very meditative man. I remember a trip that Bill and Tom took to Hawaii right before Tom died, and when they were in Hawaii, Tom became incontinent and instead of canceling the trip and bringing Tom home, Bill carried him the last week of their trip—changing diapers and carrying him all over Hawaii.

When they got back, Tom picked up the phone, called Hospice, and said, "Hello, my name is Tom and I am dying of AIDS. I don't believe that I will be here very long and what I need for you to do is come in and make me comfortable; I am in a lot of pain and, also, my lover needs some help with me." Hospice went in on a Thursday—on Friday morning another volunteer and I went in to sit with Tom because we believed that he was dying at that time, and Bill really did need some help. Tom seemed to be struggling and he had a very difficult time letting go. Toward the end of the evening I was sitting with Tom when Bill came out and said, "Irene, what's going on?" I looked up at Bill and I said, "You know, Tom is a man of rituals and what I really get from being here with him is that he needs a ritual in order to die." Bill said, "You really believe so?" I said, "Yes, why don't you put on some of that wonderful Indian music that Tom loves so much?" He said, "Oh, we have some statues and things in the closet," and I said, "Wonderful." Bill asked me, "Why don't you go out and get some food for a feast?" I said, "Okay." The other volunteer and I went out and got food for a feast.

We were gone for less than an hour. When we got back to the small apartment at the south of Market, we could hear the Indian death chant music very loudly in the streets, which let us know that Tom had died. We walked up the stairs and went into the apartment and Tom was lying out on the bed. Bill had draped the oxygen tent, removed all of the medical supplies from the room, taken rugs off the walls and put them on the floor. He had put Indian statues that they had brought back from the city of Denars, the City of the Dead, and had them lined up on a shelf all around the room and incense was burning at Tom's fingers. The other volunteer had brought silk saris and draped the bed and put flowers about and around Tom's body. The music was so beautiful, and Bill asked that we get on the phone and call people that had been in the Russian River workshop and tell them that Tom had died and we were having a feast—and that's what the other volunteer and I did.

I think one of the most beautiful things about that evening was that here was a man and his lover; the man's lover had died, and he, Bill, was allowed to openly and publicly grieve at that moment with the body, which is so important—and without reservations or formalities or being all blocked by social graces.

Another story that I remember about that evening: About ten or eleven people came and one of those people was a girlfriend of mine. She came and said, "Oh, my God, when you said Tom was here, I thought you meant in spirit. This really scares me." I asked, "What scares you about it?" She said, "What if he bites me?" So here came all those childhood scary stories that we grew up with. Well, Alice sat down and I kept assuring her that it was Tom, and that it was not scary. It was perfectly okay for her to be there, and about an hour later, she said, "I'd really like to touch it." Then I said, "Why don't you go ahead; but he's not an it, he's Tom." She said, "But I don't want to touch Tom out of love, but out of curiosity," so I said, "Well, okay, what you want to do is just scoot up and say, 'Tom, I want to touch you and it's not out of love, but it's out of curiosity.'" It took her about half an hour to scoot up close enough to talk to Tom, but she finally said, "Tom, I want to touch you and it's not out of love, it's out of curiosity," and she reached out her hand and extended her index finger and literally poked him on the foot and then made a "huh" sound when she did that.

Shortly after that, she reached over and kind of

touched him with all her fingers, and then she looked at Tom and laid her whole hand on his leg and said, "Tom, Tom, it's really you. Tom, it's really you." Then she started to pat his leg and she moved her hand up and stroked his chest and his face, and began to cry. Then she reached over and hugged him and said, "Oh, Tom, I love you so much. I'm going to miss you so much; it's really you, and it's really okay." I will never forget the feeling in me, watching someone able to openly work through the fear about death and all of the childhood horror stories about the dead rising and biting us in our sleep, and to be able to complete that relationship with Tom in his presence.

There were people in the corner crying. There were people in the kitchen eating. There were people singing around Tom. There were people moving and wailing in grief and with the rhythm. It went on until about two o'clock in the morning. It was really one of the most beautiful death experiences—it may have been one of the most beautiful life experiences that I have ever had.

We were all so very fortunate as to watch in that period of seven hours, the pain and the lines leave Tom's face. An incredible sense of peace came over his face and his lips fell into a very, very faint childlike smile, which let us know that he was not in a bad place, and we honestly got a sense that there was an energy that was traveling up from his feet and out the crown of his head and his solar plexus. We really got the sense that there was a spirit leaving his body. It was a very important experience for everyone in the room. One of the people who came was a man by the name of Peter, who had also been at the AIDS workshop. He was a K.S. patient and had a very, very serious case of it. His face was almost totally covered with

246

lesions and one of his eyes was closed. The very next morning I got a phone call from Peter, who said, "Irene, this is Peter. What you allowed me last night was one of the most remarkable experiences in my life, not to mention the most important experience so far in my illness. It gave me a sense that death is not the end, it gave me a very, very good sense of safety and peace in dying, and when I die, I want you there because I want to die in the same way."

This leads me into the story of working with Peter, and even though there are a lot of other things that I want to include, seeing that we're talking about Peter, I just want to go right into it and tell you the story. After that morning of speaking with Peter, I began to write him letters. At the Russian River workshop, there were two people that I intuitively wanted to work with. One of them was Peter and the other one was Tom.

Peter and I wrote on and off for several months and then, about six months later (what I will do is just not continue to say three months, four months, five months, six months because I have lost track of time in the year that Peter and I communicated)— One morning I was sitting at my phone when it rang. I picked it up, and the voice on the other end said, "Good morning, Irene, this is Peter," and I said, "Good morning, Peter." He said, "Irene, I'm dying," and I said, "Yes, Peter, what can I do for you?" Peter said to me, "Irene, do you know the stage in dying when all of a sudden your psyche opens out in front of you and all of your unfinished business is right there, just like an old movie going across your head?" I said, "Well, Peter, I have read about that," and he said, "Well, that's exactly where I am and I am sitting here in an enormous amount of stress and fear, and I can't put my finger on it. I don't know why I am so afraid, can you come over?" I said, "Well, yes, Peter, I can."

I got there about an hour later, and I sat down with Peter, and he said, "Irene, I have so much fear, so much fear and anger," and I said, "Peter, do you know where the anger is coming from?" He said, "Yes, I'm angry about the abuse of land and water." Peter was an extremely universal person, so I took this very seriously, in a universal way, and we talked about the abuse of land and water. He talked about his fear of leaving his friends in a world where people were rejected, instead of being a community of brothers. It scared him to leave his friends in such a world. We talked universally for a while and then we pin-pointed his personal fear, which was that he wanted to leave all of his property and the little bit of money that he had to his roommate, Tom.

He had had the same roommate for thirteen years and he was afraid that his parents would come in and they would take everything from him if his will was not legal. So after a few hours we knew that his fear was of having people rip his roommate off from what he deserved. We called a lawyer who told Peter over the phone exactly what he had to do in order to make his will legal, and they drew it up together. He wrote it out in long hand and the two of us, as witnesses, signed it. And that cleared up an enormous amount of fear for Peter.

The other fear was that he only had x amount of money and he was one hundred dollars short of having enough to be buried if he should die within the next five minutes. We got on the phone and got an instant hundred dollars so that this could be taken care of, and before the night was over, Peter was sitting and eating spaghetti in peace, with those practical fears out of the way. That night Peter sat and talked a lot about his anger about AIDS, and it was really his belief that he knew how he had contracted the AIDS virus.

I believe he said that a couple of years back, maybe in 1980, a group of men in the community was asked to be part of a hepatitis-B study, and he had volunteered. He was taken into a room where he was given an injection. He was not told what the injection was, and as he was getting the injection, the nurse said, "Oh, don't worry, we're not giving you anything that will make you sick." He said that he was told that a couple of times and that after the injection, he worried and was very sorry that he had been a part of the study. He was convinced that it was an experimentation of viruses that got out of hand. I don't know really why, but when I think of Peter this story comes to mind, so I am including it here.

During the entire year that I worked with Peter, even up until he died, he was convinced that this is how the AIDS virus, in this particular community, must have gotten some of its start. He had an enormous amount of anger about it and it seemed that, at the time he was telling me about the story, most of the people that were in this hepatitis-B study had already died of AIDS. A lot of his fear and anger came from that.

That particular evening started a very close relationship for us, and I started going over to see Peter several times a week. We did a lot of sharing and a lot of work. He finished a lot of unfinished business and our relationship allowed him to ventilate a lot of anger. He had a lot of unfinished business with his mother. She had renounced him as a person, and as a son, and then died the year before. He had a lot to work through to accept that. Peter and I became extremely close. I venture to say that it's the most incredible relationship with any human being that I have ever had in my life. I felt very much in love with Peter on all levels. He totally opened up my heart. I have never had the unconditional love inside of me opened to such a level!

The K.S. lesions started growing internally and Peter started on twenty-four-hour-a-day oxygen six months before he died. Peter said his doctor told him his lungs were about 75 percent lesions six months before he died. Peter used to tell me he could feel the lesions growing. Peter moved into a Shanti residence and began to deteriorate quite rapidly, but he never lost his love and lust for life. He was quite an extraordinary man, who absolutely refused to stay inside. Volunteers were required to take him in and out, put him in a wheelchair, and take him downstairs and outside. It was quite wonderful! I remember one day, pretty close to Christmas, when Peter called me early in the morning and said, "I feel wonderful today, Irene. I want to go to the park." So I got my neighbor and we went over to get Peter. We went inside and there was Peter all dressed. We got the portable oxygen tank, Peter, and the traveling wheelchair, and put them in the car. Then, he said, "I'll tell you what I'm going to do today. I'm going to drive!" Well, Peter had been bedridden for many months. He looked at me and said, "Irene, do you trust me to drive?"

I said, "Sure."

He asked, "Do you *really* trust me to drive?"

So I asked him, "Do *you* trust yourself to drive?"

He answered, "Yes"; so I said, "Okay, I trust you to drive."

To which Peter replied, "Okay, I'll tell you what I want you to do. I want you and Andy to take me south of

Market to where my van is parked and don't worry about any of this as I have cab fare in my pocket. You two take me out there where my van is and I'll get in it and you get in with me. So what we're going to do is I'll drive for a couple of blocks and Andy can drive behind us. If I find out that I can't drive, then we can stop, and Andy can get into the van and drive back to the parking lot. If I find out that I can drive, we'll just keep driving and Andy can go on home. If I start getting sick, or I can't make it, what I'll do is, I will pull over to the side of the road. Don't worry about a thing, Irene, I have cab fare. I have a pocket full of money today."

I said, "Okay, Peter."

You have to understand that Peter was extremely ravished by K.S. One of the most severe cases that I have seen. One of his eyes had been radiated; granted, the lesions on the eye had disappeared, but the eye had closed due to the radiation. Occasionally, it was open so that there was just a little bit of a slit through which he could see, but most of the time it was completely covered over. So there was Peter and his one eye, and his little bedridden body, and he was going to drive that great big old van. So off the three of us went! Well, we got south of Market and I've got to tell you that my downstairs neighbor was a nervous wreck! When we got to the van, Andy said, "Irene, I can't leave you in that van with Peter," and I said, "Oh, sure you can." Andy said, "No, I can't! I'm going to leave my car here and if the three of us will get into the van, we can let Peter drive a couple of blocks and if we see that he can't drive, I'll take over the wheel." I said, "Okay."

We got in the van and I wish you could have been there! Peter got in that big old wide van, turned up the country and western music, put his arm out the window, and started driving. He got so excited that he started jumping up and down on the seat and waving to people. He waved to all the trucks that passed him, and said, "Look at me; my name's Peter. I'm supposed to be dead and I'm driving." We laughed, we got excited, and he jumped up and down and drove!

Peter was an outpatient of Ward 86 at San Francisco General Hospital, and what he wanted to do was drive over to the hospital and pick up his medication. During the whole time he was driving, he had the country and western music up and was waving to the people on the street. It is one of those days that lights me up to talk about it and it will be in my heart forever. We got to Ward 86 and he started hollering out the window to all the people from the hospital . . . walking by, "Look at me, look at me, I'm driving, I'm driving. I have AIDS and I'm supposed to be dead." He sent me into the pharmacy to get his medication. I came back with the medication, and he said, "I think I'm a little pooped now, I'll let Andy drive." . . . The next few minutes were taken up with Peter's excitement over having driven—just hardly believing it. Then the three of us drove off. That was quite an exciting day! Peter insisted on having ice cream, juice, apples, and bananas, so at every little store we saw we stopped and got something to eat.

He asked if we would drive by his home where he had lived for thirteen years before he moved into the Shanti residence. He had been a stained-glass worker and all of his belongings were in that house. We helped him out of the van and up on the front porch so he could visit with his cats—one of them, Moon-gold, he had had for eight years. One of us had to walk right behind Peter with the portable oxygen on our shoulders. We all got seated on the front porch and he started calling the cats. When he called, "Kitty, kitty," the cats were a little bit scared. It was very difficult for him to get near them, and at one point I had tears in my eyes and thought, "Oh, God, please let the cats come and say 'good-bye.'" Peter sat on the porch and he finally coaxed Moon-gold onto his lap and talked to her. He told her how much he loved her and how much he missed her. Then he cried and told Moon-gold good-bye.

We were there for about fifteen minutes when Peter said, "Okay, I'm ready to go to the park." The three of us got into the van and went out to Golden Gate Park, where he wanted to go to his very, very favorite spot, which was a hill with a waterfall and a little lake with ducks. Now you've got to understand that it was the middle of a very hot sunny afternoon, and the park was filled with senior citizens and all kinds of little ladies taking their afternoon walks. We got out the wheelchair, the oxygen, and put Peter in the wheelchair and started wheeling him through the park. He stopped and looked at the flowers, the trees, the ducks, and he stopped and talked to every little lady walking through the park. He would say, "Hello, my name is Peter, isn't it a beautiful day!" It *was* a beautiful day! (When I had met Peter at the AIDS workshop in 1983, his mattress work was anger with Mother Earth, and as he beat the phone books, he cursed Mother Earth for what she had done to him and to his brothers.) As we were wheeling past the hill that day in the park, he said, "Oh, stop, I want to lie in the grass." So we stopped the wheelchair and I took a blanket and my jacket and put them on the grass, and Peter crawled on his stomach onto the grass.

I sat down and, at first, he put his head in my lap. Then he asked me to move and he put his face into the grass and lay there for quite some time, and the afternoon chill came. Since Peter had pneumocystis, I began to worry about the chill, so I mentioned it to him and he said, "No, leave me alone, don't worry, I'm not getting chilled, I just want to lie here." Peter lay there and talked to Mother Earth, made peace with her, and told her that he understood that it was not her fault, that he loved her, and that it was okay. When he had finished, we got him up and put him in the wheelchair, then we wheeled him back to the van. We got into the van, and he said, "Okay, I want to see the ocean." We drove to the ocean by way of the ice-cream store and the apple-pie store.

At the ocean, Andy got out for a couple of minutes while Peter and I sat in the van. He turned the country and western music up a little louder. He didn't say a word, just sat and listened to the ocean. We would look at each other and smile, and he would say, "Oh, God, Irene, isn't it a beautiful day. I feel fantastic! I feel fantastic, isn't it a beautiful day!" The sun started to go down and it was time to go home, so we drove Peter back to the Shanti residence and took him back up the stairs. I gave Peter a kiss and told him I would see him later. It was, indeed, a beautiful day!

I want to go back a little, to when Peter first moved into the Shanti residence. He had been living at home on twenty-four-hour-a-day oxygen, and it had come to a point where he really did need more care than his roommate, Joe, was able to provide. Joe's life had been rather upside down for the past two years, actually three years, of Peter's illness. To have Hospice come in with the attendants and for the level of care that Peter was going to need at that point in time, we decided that what he would need to do was to move into a residence home. After checking one out, Peter decided that Shanti would be a very good place for him to finish out his illness. So he moved into a Shanti residence. The second day he was there I went over to visit him and I gave him a massage. It was a new residence home, and there was only one other gentleman there, at the end of the hall, and he had twenty-four-hour-a-day maintenance care because he had gone blind and was totally bedridden. I really didn't understand that the attendant care was basically for the other gentleman; I was under the assumption that Peter did have twenty-four-hour care, and that he was okay.

About a week later I had a massage appointment with Peter and I arrived at the Shanti residence when another one of his friends also arrived there. His other friend had a key and when we went in, we walked down to Peter's room and he was sitting in a chair, very panicked, very anxiety-ridden, and he was rather humped in the chair and not breathing very well. It seemed that Peter had been alone in the house over the weekend—this was on a Monday. He had been alone on Saturday and Sunday except for a four-hour attendant who came in to clean and prepare his meals. Other than that, he had been alone, and what we found was Peter trying to dial the phone and unable to do so because he was so stricken. In his words, he had been suffocating for a couple of days, without any help. I asked Peter if he would like to go to the hospital and he said no, but he wanted me to stay with him, and he asked his other friend to leave. His friend left, and I asked Peter again if he would like to go to the hospital, and he said, "No, Irene. I believe that you can handle this and just be with me." It was quite an evening and one that I will never forget!

Peter was, on some level, suffocating and he would grab his chest and try to breathe, but was unable to do so. He couldn't really walk more than one or two steps and then he had to bend over from the waist and hold on to something. All night long he went from the bed to the chair, from the chair to the bed, the bed to the chair. I sat all night and talked to him. There were many times during the night when Peter and I both thought he was dying and that this would be it, but he still preferred not to go to the hospital.

I think one of the most important things I learned that evening was the power of the relaxing voice, the power of the breath, and breathing with a person who is in pain, connecting with that person, and, with our breath, flowing as one. It was a very important experience for me, for Peter, and for my work. When morning came, I got on the phone, called the Hospice, and stated that I was in a Shanti residence with Peter whom I had found alone, sitting in a chair, suffocating, and that he definately needed twenty-four-hour-a-day attendant care. What had happened was that when Peter had moved into the Shanti residence, he was assessed as needing four-hour-a-day care. He had deteriorated and had reached an extreme level of anxiety since he had been in the house because it was a very difficult move for him. He had not been reassessed since his move, so at that time, he did not have the proper care. I was told that the nurse would come over and assess the situation.

Since it was daylight, Peter said that he would like to go to the hospital and see if they could help him breathe. He asked me not to leave him, so I promised I would not.

The nurse came over. I stayed with Peter and sat right down on the floor next to his bed, holding his hand, looking into his eyes and breathing with him. It was at that time that Peter and I definitely became as one and it started a bonding unlike any I have ever known with another person. The ambulance came. Peter asked me to ride with him in the ambulance, and when we got to Ward 86, which was the outpatient clinic for people with AIDS, he wanted me to talk to the doctor and tell him what was going on with him because he didn't really feel like he could explain it. He wanted me to let the doctor know what I had found out about his suffocating, and that he needed twenty-four-hour-a-day care. He also wanted me to let the doctors know that, if this was it, he wanted to be a "No Code," which simply means no life-saving machines, no life-saving devices; he wanted to go in a natural way. Also, he wanted to be at home with twenty-four-hour-a-day care.

He asked me to stay with him because he was afraid they would do a lot of different painful procedures on him that he really didn't want, and if I were there, he would not be taken through all the examinations that he had before. So that's what I did. I talked to the people in 86. We were admitted into General; we were not able to get on 5B, but we did get on the fourth floor at about five o'clock that afternoon. When we went into the room, a Shanti volunteer was there who asked me if there was anything I needed and I said, "Yes, what I need to do is to go home, feed the cats, and get some fresh clothes, if I am going to stay in the hospital again tonight," so the Shanti volunteer sat with Peter, who made me promise to come back.

I promised him that I would be back and went home

257

for about an hour. I returned to the hospital and Peter had already been taken to Xray. He was coming up the hall and was encircled by three Shanti volunteers. We all got back to the room and Peter really believed that he was in the process of dying, and he was telling the volunteers good-bye. He also had one of the volunteers call his roommate and tell him that he really wasn't needed there, but this really might be it. At about 11:00 P.M. everyone left. The nurse let me know that, though there was no cot on the floor, I could stay in with Peter, so I sat up with him all night. Peter didn't talk much, but I sat next to him all night long and held his hand. We breathed together and looked into each other's eyes, and once again I was made aware of the power of the breath, the power of love, the power of clarity, and being connected with another human being. One of the scenes that stays in my mind, when I'm going over the entire year with Peter, happened that night. He had a very short oxygen tube and the tube was attached to the wall. At one point he wanted to look down the hallway, so he scooted to the end of the bed and sat, but he really couldn't sit where he could see down the hallway. So there was this man covered with K.S. lesions, humped over, somewhat like the hunchback of Notre Dame, attached to that oxygen tube, one eye totally closed, trying to peek around the room and down the hallway. For some reason that picture has stuck in my heart and in my mind. I didn't say anything, and neither did Peter; he just kept looking and peeking around like a little animal of some sort. He was really assessing his life at that point and he was assessing the quality of his life. He told me that later.

The next day, at 7:00 A.M., I did leave, and he was assessed as needing twenty-four-hour-a-day care and sent back to the Shanti residence. At that point there were not enough funds for Peter to have twenty-four-hour-a-day attendant care. (This has been one of the biggest challenges of people with AIDS: the fact that they need so much care and there just aren't enough funds.) You know, our senior citizens usually reach a level of deterioration and then they die. What happens to people with AIDS is that they reach a level of deterioration and they continue to live. They really *do* need twenty-four-hour-a-day care.

I was told on the phone by the Shanti house manager that if Peter could not find twenty-four-hour-a-day care he would be asked to leave the residence, as they were not able to handle him. So what happened was there was a group of about seven of Peter's friends and I who got together and made a schedule of each one taking on an eight-hour shift—one person each day—and attendance care covered the rest. So the attendants and a circle of friends took care of Peter. His friends came in the evenings and cooked dinner for him, and so Peter was very well taken care of at the Shanti residence. The only thing that really panicked Peter, and was where most of his anxiety came from, was the fact that due to the K.S. lesions in his lungs he had feelings of suffocation, and became extremely afraid of the dark.

The attendants that were on in the evenings went through that every day with Peter, and two of them who became very close to him were willing to sit up and talk to him at night. (The level of attendant care in this situation really, really needs to be [addressed.] There are so few attendants who are clear enough of their own fears and anxieties who can cope with taking care of AIDS patients. This is a very sad situation. Attendants are having to be hired so fast with such low funds, there just isn't proper training. They do not have support groups, and there is no place for them to go for help or for [venting] their [own] emotions. This is very sad because the patient is the one who takes the brunt of it. The attendant makes about 80 percent of the patient's atmosphere in his process of dying, most especially the patient who doesn't have a family with him twenty-four hours a day. . . . There should be a lot of concern with training and hiring attendants and it just isn't there. The time limit with people who are getting sick is short, the funds are low, and people who are available to take care of them are too few. This needs to be changed.)

Peter had an enormous amount of anxiety because he was constantly under the care of strangers, and a lot of the attendants even voiced fears about being with people with AIDS, but they were there because they needed the money.

Spending the night with Peter at the Shanti residence became a routine, and it was a very rewarding routine for me. I loved Peter very, very much and I looked forward to the evenings we spent together. A lot of times he was afraid of the attendants that were in the house, so I would go over and stay with him. I spoiled him rotten, and if I had the chance, I would do it all over again! He was worth it. We became like brother and sister. When daylight would come, I would leave and Peter would be okay. I've talked about the story of that wonderful afternoon in the park, and now I will tell you about Christmas with Peter.

Eventually, Peter had an enormous amount of love and support in the Shanti residence. He had his Shanti volunteers, the attendants, and a circle of friends. [But he dreamed of going] home for Christmas; he wanted to be with his cats again, he wanted to be in the house where his things were, and he wanted to be with his roommate during Christmas. We all had a feeling that Peter was hanging on so that he could be in his own home during Christmas. Peter's spirits were up and down, but basically, he had an enormous passion for life and a very enlightened spirit, and, therefore, he really did have quite a bit of energy.

We made plans to take Peter home for Christmas. About two days before Christmas, Peter had a couple of seizures in a row. I was called and told that he was dying, and [asked if I wanted] to come and be with him. I went to the Shanti residence, and I tell you the truth, I really didn't feel like he would make it till Christmas. Well, bless his heart, the next morning, he woke up, looked at everybody and said, "Now don't just stand there, let's get ready for Christmas!"

On Christmas Eve day we had to find three people to carry the wheelchair, with Peter in it, down the stairs. (Until this point, when he had left the house, he would crawl down the stairs and we would put him in the wheelchair, but he was not able to crawl up or down the stairs now.) Also, we needed to pack up a multitude of nursing equipment [so he could] spend the night at home. So on Christmas Eve day I found three Shanti volunteers who were willing to pack him up and move him home. The attendant showed me all the things I would need to know to take care of Peter for the evening and through the next day: giving him his medication, using the bedpan and urinal, working his oxygen unit, giving him his bed bath, doctoring his sores, and doing his mouth care. The Shanti volunteers came and we got Peter dressed. The three volunteers carried seven boxes of equipment down to a cab that I had called, and then carried Peter down the stairs to his wheelchair. I would give anything on God's green earth to have a picture of that!

The cab driver asked me what was wrong with him and I said, "Well, the man has AIDS." Immediately I thought, "Oh, no, the cab driver is going to have a level of fear," but he said to me, "Oh, I'm gay, this will be a wonderful experience for me." God bless San Francisco, it's quite a city!

When Peter came down the front stairs of the building in his wheelchair, he looked at me and then at the cab driver, and said, "What's the matter, haven't you ever seen Cleopatra?" Peter had an incredible sense of humor. We got him in the cab and folded up the wheelchair. There we were with four people plus Peter and seven boxes of equipment. We could hardly see out the cab windows, but we were on our way to Larkin Street. When we got out, I went to pay the cab driver and he looked at me and said, "Oh, no, thank you so much. God bless you, and have a Merry Christmas." Peter never forgot that. On his deathbed, he remembered the cab driver that had given him that Christmas present and he said, "That cab driver is blessed." It meant a lot to Peter.

We got to Peter's house, and we went up the stairs and his roommate had everything ready. The house was all decorated—there was a gorgeous tree with all the Christmas ornaments Peter's had gathered over the years—and we went into a very comfortable living room where Peter was able to lie on his sofa. His dream was to sleep on a mattress under the Christmas tree with me, so . . . we put a mattress under the Christmas tree, and then two volunteers went home.

One volunteer and I got Peter on the mattress underneath the tree and the volunteer sat up all night long wrapping Christmas presents, with Christmas music playing and Peter lying there looking at the Christmas tree. I will never forget that Christmas. It was the most beautiful Christmas I have ever had in my life. At about two o'clock in the morning, the volunteer went home. I put on my pajamas and crawled onto the mattress next to Peter. And the most incredible thing about Peter, that I will always remember, when spending the night with him, was that he would wake up every couple of hours, and ask, "Irene, are you okay?" I would say, "Yes, Peter, I'm okay," and he would say, "Okay, I can go to sleep now." Every couple of hours he would wake me up and ask me if I was okay.

Peter had been having nights of anxiety, and had been throwing up in the night, but that night he didn't need a tranquilizer, he didn't wake up in anxiety, and he didn't throw up. I got up quite early on Christmas morning and put all the presents under the tree. I got myself ready and a few hours later Peter woke up and I did his mouth and sore care, gave him his bath and dressed him, and put him on the living room sofa. Then I put the mattress away and made the room ready for visitors. . . . His roommate got up and started fixing the turkey.

Friends stopped by throughout the day. Peter's friends came by and exchanged presents and it was just a really extraordinary day. It was such a thrill to be a part of knowing that with volunteer help and a little nursing instruction, Peter was allowed to carry out one of his very, very deepest wishes, and that was to spend Christmas at home with his roommate, his cats, and [surrounded by his own] things. Volunteers mean so much, and as volunteers, we get to help patients really give quality to their lives in their dying processes, and that is very, very important—not to mention the light that it puts in our hearts.

I guess it was about seven o'clock in the evening—and mind you, this was Christmas night—when Peter told us to call the volunteers, he needed to go [back to the residence]. We called the same volunteers. They came over; we packed Peter's stuff, put him in a cab, and took him back to the Shanti residence. When we got there, Peter was quite pooped. One of the attendants had rented the video of *Gandhi* for him because one of Peter's wishes was to see that film. Frank was a very special attendant [and he] meant a lot to Peter and he would spend many, many nights up with Peter. . . . I'd really like to acknowledge him at this point for his work with Peter. It was very, very wonderful. Peter asked me if I would watch the movie with him, so we lay in bed on this night and we watched *Gandhi* until about one o'clock in the morning. When Peter drifted off to sleep, I went home. Ah, Christmas 1984—one of the most memorable Christmases of my life, and what a bright light in my heart!

All of us had a feeling that Peter would let go pretty soon after Christmas, but this really didn't come about. Peter lived until January 17. Very early in our relationship, Peter had asked that when he died, I be with him. . . . What he wanted was that when he died, he wanted me to be alone in the room with him, and for me to get up and close the door and sit with him for anywhere from three to eight hours during the first part of his transition and make sure that his body was undisturbed, and that no one else came into the room. He felt that I had the experience to do that without panicking. It was his wish that I be with him when he died, and, of course, I told him, "Yes, I will be with you."

His wishes were that [during this] three- to eight-hour period I would get on my knees and pray to Jesus that He "carry this boy home." He wanted me to tell Jesus all the wonderful things about him, and that he was on his way home, and for Him to hold him and guide him gently. In the second week of January, another one of Peter's wishes was that if he reached a point where he could not respond, he did not want to be heavily medicated. It was his wish that he die a conscious death. He believed that he would be able to work through more things if he were conscious. I reached a point where I needed about a week away from this situation. My roommate was moving and I needed some time to myself, so I did not see Peter for a week.

When I went back to the Shanti residence to see Peter, he was unable to talk, he was unable to communicate, he could not move and his eyes were very big, and he looked to be in an enormous amount of pain. I didn't quite understand what was going on with him, but I sat with him until about four o'clock in the morning and he was screaming, "Oh Jesus, oh Jesus," and he was in an extreme level of anxiety and pain. I was with him for the next four days and his condition did not change. However, I did notice that the attendant would come in every three hours and give him Dilaudid suppositories for pain. I knew that it was Peter's wish not to be medicated to that point. I noticed that about three hours after he would get his suppositories, he would be calm. The panic and horror started when the suppository was given again, which led me to believe that he was having morphine hallucinations. I got extremely angry, I didn't quite know what to do. I talked with the other attendant, Frank, and he said, "Yes, Peter was getting extremely high doses of Dilaudid suppositories."

At this point Peter had been in bed for several days

without even being able to have any water, his mouth was open, he was in pain, filled with horror and anxiety. When the nurse came over one evening, I asked her if she could please drive me around the block. We went for a drive around the block and I told her that she had better roll up the windows. She rolled up the windows. I stomped the floor of the car, I screamed and hollered, I beat the seats, and I told her that what was going on was not right, that a hospice was supposed to stand for dignity, control, and quality of life, but what was in that bed was not of any quality and did not express dignity or control.

I told her that Peter's wishes were [that he not be] heavily medicated to the point where he could not respond, that he wanted a conscious death, and that the medication needed to be stopped. She assured me that he was not getting a high dose of suppositories. I told her that what she needed to do was to check the chart! That attendant had been giving such and such a dosage, and with another medication. Another attendant would give him two, another would give him three, and still another attendant would give him one, so what we had was somebody being bounced up and down on all different levels of medication. Peter was in an enormous amount of pain and stress, and something had to be done about the attendant care. She came over, picked up the notebook that the attendants kept, and went home.

About an hour later, she called me and said, "I believe you are right. I've been thinking about it, and if it's Peter's wishes that he not be medicated at this point, then we do not need to medicate him." The suppositories were discontinued. However, during this period of medication, Peter had deteriorated to a very high degree. He [lived only another] three days. As soon as the medication went down, he began to run extremely high fevers and we took turns, along with the attendants, keeping Peter in cold cloths, wiping him down, and being with him. I stayed with him for five nights in a row. I slept next to him. I told him I had never had anyone trust me as much, and it was an honor to give our relationship to God because it was a relationship that was worthy of Heaven, and when I said those words to Peter he really responded with his whole body. It was a loving release. His eyes were wide open, he was panting as if he were running around the block, his mouth open.

On the fifth day of this, the nurse came by. At this point in the dying cycle, everyone is always trying to figure out what they can do to help the patient let go. [They wonder] why it's taking so long, and they will do things like sit around the bed and say, "Just let go, just let go." The nurse said that possibly why Peter couldn't let go was that I was hanging on to him so much, maybe I needed to go away so that he could let go, and I thought, "Well, maybe this is correct," so I went in and told Peter that I was going to go home for a little while, and if he wanted to let go while I was gone, it would be okay.

I went home and I sat on the deck and looked at the sky. A little voice told me, "Irene, Peter wants you there," so I simply returned and I went into the room and I was with him until about eight o'clock in the evening. On and off, there were about seven or eight other people who were there also. One of Peter's other friends, Jim had been there doing shifts in the daytime while I would go out and take care of patients. On this particular evening, Jim, asked, "Do you think it is okay if I go home?" I said, "Yes, I do. I'll be here all night." Jim left and there were about four or five people in the room. We turned Peter.

Turning was so painful for him, he gritted his teeth. After that, everyone left the room except me.

I sat on the bed next to Peter and put my hand on his shoulders and I noticed that he was really looking through me—right through me—and he had such an incredible determined look on his face, somewhat like an Indian chief—an Indian chief who knew he was going to win the war—and while looking through me, all of a sudden his little body started shaking and it started letting go. My heart started to pound a little bit and I said to myself, "It's perfectly okay, Irene," and Peter's bowels let go, his other body fluids let go, and then he looked at me—straight through me—and took his lips and shut his mouth making a very square chin, and with total determination, held his breath while looking into my eyes. I just looked down and kept saying "Good, Peter, good, yes, yes, that's it, good." I waited only a couple of minutes, then I went over and turned off the oxygen and took off the oxygen mask.

Peter's other wish was that, in sitting with him, at no time was I to shed tears because he believed tears would bog down the spirit. It was at the time that I took off the oxygen mask and when his body had let go, his other eye had opened and both of those eyes were looking straight through me. I thought, "Will I really be able to sit here without grieving?" I put the oxygen mask away, I got up and shut the door, and I sat back down—my heart pounding and my mind thinking that I must have [a million things to do,] but my little intuitive voice [told] me that I didn't have to do a thing but just sit there in the quiet and be with Peter. I sat for a few moments, then I got up and walked out of the room. I let the attendant and the other volunteer in the house know that Peter was in transition and I told them that I would be going back in the room and would be sitting with him for eight hours.

I put on some very gentle, spiritual breathing music, then I sat down on the bed and lit some candles and some incense. Peter had pictures of Jesus, and he had this one particular picture of Him that he had taken from the hospital, to his house, to the Shanti residence, everywhere he went. That picture of Jesus always had to be with him, and at one point, when he was unable to respond and was lying in bed, people had taken that picture and taped it to the wall to [where he could see it] when he was turned. So I took the picture of Jesus, his pictures of St. Francis, the incense, and I made a little altar on the table beside his bed. Then I got down on my knees and I began to pray out loud for Jesus to come and carry "His boy home"; that Peter was knocking at the door and he needed guidance and a guiding light. I continued to pray for Peter to stay in the light and stay focused in the light. I also told Jesus that Peter was a good man, a creative man, that he had loved and given to his friends; he was a very fine artist, and that he had given the world his love and his creative talents and that even though Peter had studied many rituals, his heart belonged to Jesus and now he was coming home.

I shall never forget that night, on my knees next to Peter in transition, saying those prayers out loud. Every few moments, I would feel a wave of grief coming, and what would go through my mind was that my earthly relationship with Peter had changed, and the words that came to me eased and helped me with the transition that I was going through at that point, being in that room and being with Peter in this stage of life, I felt that I was not losing Peter but that we were simply having a relationship on a different level. When the tears would start to come, my mind would say all kinds of things to keep them down, and I would say words like joy, peace, light, radiance, harmony, and freedom. "Joy, peace, radiance, harmony, light, and freedom," and the tears would subside for I knew that I had promised Peter that I would not cry. I prayed for about two hours and I have to say that it became like a mantra to Jesus, and there was such a presence of life and reverence and light in the room during that period!

I don't have the words for it, but it was like being in a House of God. Everything was soft, but pulsating and radiant. All of a sudden I would look at Peter, and say, "Yoo hoo, are you in there?" "Are you doing okay?" "Yoo hoo, how're you doing?" Yes, that was a bit of humor, and I know, also, that it was my way of not letting Peter go. I kept acknowledging the fact that he was in there and, at one point, I finally said, "Well, Peter, you will know it anyway, but I have to leave the room and smoke," and that's just what I did. I left the room, had a couple of cigarettes, some dinner, and then I went back into the room.

It had been Peter's wish that I bathe his body, but not really disturb it. What I found was that Peter's weight was such that I really couldn't turn him and bathe his sores without really creating a lot of movement with his body and I knew he wouldn't want that, so I let him know that I would get the attendant and the other volunteer, sitting out in the living room and who would sit there all night, to come in around daylight and we would bathe his body before Neptune [funeral service] would pick him up. After dinner, when I went back into the room and told Peter this, I looked at him and I thought to myself, "Jesus, you know, I just want to lie down and put my arms around Peter and go to sleep and have this one last nap with him," and that's what I did.

I lay down and snuggled up real close and when I did this, I looked at Peter and sensed that while I was on watch for, oh, about four hours now, all of his past was coming over him. I honestly saw a pharaoh in him and I also saw an Indian chief. I will never forget the squared jaw of the pharaoh and the determination in that square jaw, also the ease and peace and strength that came over his face. At one point, I really know that I was looking at a Saint Peter; the lines left his face, the lesions lightened, the look of peace and radiance came over his face, and when I lay next to him, I felt that I was lying in strength and power and I put my arm around Peter and my head on his shoulder. When I did this I heard this little voice in me say, "Irene, you need to let Peter go. It's okay to lie here, but why not back off a little and let him go on with his transition?" So that's what I did. I scooted over just a couple of inches, because I wanted to be so close, and fell into the most peaceful and deep sleep.

I had told the attendant and volunteer that I would wake them up at about 4:30 A.M. so I could bathe his body, and what happened was, all of a sudden, I realized that I was above Peter and me. I looked down at us—I looked at Peter and then looked at me, and I said, "Irene, Peter's dead and it's time to bathe his body." I put my feet on the floor, got out of bed, and walked into the other room. I got the attendant and the volunteer, and we took a very large pan of water and sandalwood incense soap and went into the bedroom where we bathed Peter's body. We took the bandages off his sores and dressed them. It was at that point that we gave ourselves permission to grieve and we did. We talked to him and we cried and cried. I held him and I cried and cried, and we washed him with our tears. Then we washed him with the soap and what an incredible thing it was to be able to go through that level of grief together—with the body—and also to know that we had fulfilled this man's wishes in death. He was allowed total dignity and control in his transition and, God, how wonderful it feels that this was carried out.

I have to tell you that in the middle of the evening the nurse called and said they wanted to pick up the body. We really had seen to it that his wishes were enforced and that he lay there the way he wanted to, and, oh, God, that's so important. We got Peter's body bathed and all cleaned up, and then, one by one, we spent a little more time with him. When it was daylight, his very favorite time, and the birds were chirping, Neptune came with a stretcher and a gorgeous red cloth. They took Peter's body from the bed and wrapped it in the most beautiful vibrant red cloth and then laid a little strap across it. We put flowers, fresh white daisies, under the strap on top of the red wrapping, and Peter's body was carried off in the daylight with the birds chirping.

The other volunteer took me home, and as I walked up my stairs I thought, "This is going to be hard, I have been with Peter for so long." From my bedroom there are sliding glass doors that go up to a deck that overlooks a lot of trees, often with many little birds in them. My bed is right where the sliding glass doors are. When I walked in it was about 7:30 A.M. I looked out and saw that the deck was covered with birds. There were birds all over the floor of the deck, and there were birds right up against each other all along the railing. There were hundreds of birds! My deck was almost solid birds and my two cats were lying on the bed looking out at them. Even though the sliding glass doors were open, their little heads were draped over the bed just looking at the birds with love, and I knew it was okay.

I sat and looked in wonderment and I shed tears of joy and grief, petting the cats and looking at the birds. When I walked into my kitchen I heard a sound, a very strong sound of a very strong bird in the house, and I looked on my cats' catwalk, which is a board that goes from my hallway window to the roof, and there was a huge blue jay standing right on the walk inside the window looking at me, singing cheerfully, and I said, "Good morning, Peter." I love this story!

About two weeks later we had a service for Peter. We went out on the very highest point of Twin Peaks, which is a beautiful view here in the city, because this was where Peter wanted us to scatter his ashes. We went to this peak and we climbed way up and stood in a little circle, and each person shared what he wanted to share about his relationship with and about Peter. It was a gorgeous sunny day and there was a beautiful breeze. Then we went to the farthest side of the point and threw the ashes, and when it was over there was maybe a third of the box of ashes left so we poured all of them into the lid of the box and we went dancing all around the hill scattering the whole box of ashes, and people would say things like, "Peter, we love you." It was a very, very moving service, after which we had a wake over at my house where we just all got together, talked about Peter, and ate turkey and listened to a type of Eastern music that Peter like to hear. God bless Peter!

Another one of my fondest memories about this work is that I had decided that I was going to have a yoga class for people with AIDS. So I had a yoga class in my bedroom and there were four students. One day one of them, George, called up and said, "Irene, I am having extreme liver pain, I'm throwing up, and I have diarrhea. I really don't feel well and what I would really like to do is take a cab and come over," and I said, "Of course, George, come on over." George came right over. As I opened the cab door for him he said, "Please, I've got to run upstairs, I have to lie down fast. My liver's killing me." I said, "Okay." So he ran upstairs and lay down on the living room floor. The other three students were already there, and we went over to George and all laid our hands on him stroking him gently, and we did a little relaxation for him and talked to him about relaxing and being easy with the pain, and pretty soon George said, "Well, I'm ready to do a little yoga," so we all gathered around the floor and started doing yoga.

All of a sudden we looked over at George, who was very, very deteriorated and had had all these problems with his liver earlier in the day, and he was standing on his head with his feet straight up in the air, and I said, "George, I'm a little worried about you doing that," and he said, "Don't worry, Irene, it makes me feel great." . . . When he came down, he looked at me and said, "Oh, don't worry, Irene, when I die, I'll come back and help you with your yoga." He added, "I know you can't do a head stand, so I'll come back and pull you up by your feet!" Ah, anyway, that was a real special day.

We finished our yoga class. I did a couple of massages, and then George decided that he wanted to go to the health food store and buy groceries so I said, "Okay." . . . I'll never understand how he got [those huge bags of groceries] back to the house and up three flights of stairs! Then he came in and said, "I'm really pooped, I'd like a massage," and I said, "Great." George was covered with lesions and was very, very thin. About an hour into the massage, he let me know that he had not been touched in about a year. George was known all over the world. He was one of the best-looking men that I have ever seen, and the most incredible thing about him was his dignity and his pride. He looked like a model until the day he died. He never lost his sense of dignity. His heart only grew, and on top of all this dignity and all this pride, he had unconditional love coming from every part of his body.

We did a massage and [when we finished George said something that] I'll never forget. He said, "You know, Irene, if I die tonight, I know that I'm a whole, perfect, beautiful, radiant being and I know that I am loved." I will never forget that. It was one of the most touching things that anyone has ever said to me. George and I went into the hallway and we talked for a little bit and he said he needed to go home, he had been here all day long, and he lived in a Shanti residence, so I said, "Okay," and called us a cab. We were about four or five blocks from the Shanti residence when George told the cab driver he was going to have to stop. The cab driver stopped and George walked around the side of the cab, right on the street, and he walked over behind another car and started throwing up. He threw up again and again. I asked the cab driver if he had a Kleenex or something and he said he didn't. So I looked in George's bag and found one of his diapers which I had given him and he wiped his face and the front of his shirt with it. Then he looked at me and said, "Okay, I'm ready." We got back in the cab. He looked at the cab driver and said, "Thank you so much, I feel much better." When we got to the Shanti residence, the cab driver helped him with his groceries, and George gave him a big kiss and said, "Thank you so much, I'll see you later."

About three days after that I got a phone call saying that George was in a very, very serious condition, and he was going back to Denver. It was his choice to go back and die at home with his parents, so I went over to the Shanti residence to say good-bye. I went in while the attendant was packing his clothes and George was lying on the mattress. We sat and talked and talked about how much fun we had had. He talked about how he had gone to an externalization workshop, and how that was the greatest healing that he had ever had in his life; how getting rid of his anger and his feelings about getting AIDS and about people having always used him and how he had longed for love and really never found it. He said the experience of being able to work all that out at the workshop was the most important experience during his illness and one of the most important experiences of his life. He talked about being able to find love and to come in contact with that space of love inside himself because of that workshop.

George and I had a couple of hours that day, and it was wonderful. He used to collect jewels; so he took a couple of jewels out and gave me one and said, "Now, Irene, I'll tell you what I want you to do. I want you to put this little stone on your dresser and I want you to look at it every day, and one day when you walk by this jewel it will be shining brightly just like the sun, and you will know that I am sitting on your dresser, so just tell me, 'Hello.' "

George went back to Denver and I communicated with his parents. He was in ICU for two weeks before he died. I wrote his parents several letters; I never did get a response, but I just know that they are okay, and I certainly know that George is okay. And I have that little jewel, but you know, I don't have it on my dresser, and I haven't looked for it, so I think I will do that now.

Working with people with AIDS as much as I do, people are constantly dying around me. My friends are constantly dying. I experienced seventy-four deaths in the last year or the past year and a half, so I am in the constant process of grief, and about the first year that I worked like this I found that watching one's friends die every day can probably be an extremely horrible experience and one can really click into the pain and horror of it. AIDS is such a visual disease and one is constantly faced with such a level of helplessness and deterioration that it can seemingly be quite horrible, and then one day you will be sitting in a hospital with someone who is dying, and all of a sudden you look around and you've got seven or eight volunteers in the room and you are all touching each other and you're all holding hands and being with each other and you notice that the most incredible, positive thing is going on. You're sitting in the midst of what life is really supposed to be all about, and that is loving, caring, supporting, and sharing with one another. People ask me all the time, "How can you do this, it's so depressing?" I have to tell them that it is not, that it is the most joyful time in my life to be involved on such a level of unconditional love and support. It only makes your heart unfold and it brings light into your life. It affords you an opportunity to do an enormous amount of work on yourself, for that's what this work is. It is working on yourself. It's working through your fears, anger, doubts, and insecurities about life and coming in contact with that space inside of us that is pure unconditional love, and when this love enters your life, your life turns into one of radiance and joy. It's what life is all about. People are always trying to get me to go to a movie or a party, or something like that.

Sometimes I sit in a group of people who aren't connected with this work and they are standing quite a bit of distance away from each other and they are holding things in their hands, talking fast, and their eyes are going one way, then another, and they are talking about cars, new clothes, and I think, "God, how wonderful it is to sit at the hospital with a group of people that are sitting close, touching one another, and talking about things that have to do with love, with feelings, and with life, and having to do with growth and opportunity, and I think, "This is living." And so I have to say, "No, it is not depressing for me to go to the hospital or the Shanti residence or be with people who are dying, because it's being with people who are actually living. It means that you have to keep your own feelings very well ventilated and up to date so that you can constantly deal with what is real, and you're constantly dealing with yourself and others and you know how to reach out in love, care, and support for one another. Why else are we on this planet? By reaching out, loving, communicating, and supporting one another, that's how we will heal this planet."

I honestly believe that AIDS is a healing of our time. I believe it's where our teachers are being taught at this time and the teachers in love and in healing that are coming out of the AIDS epidemic will be some of the greatest teachers that we've ever had. It's at this time that I would like to acknowledge the gay community in our country that has rallied and gotten together and formed such an incredible circle of support around its own, as the gay community in San Francisco. To be a part of what is going on here is real history. Everyone is growing, everybody is reaching out to all different types . . . and forms of healing due to the fact that one's friends are constantly dying around one in this community. Everybody is working on oneself and clearing the space to be with people; clearing a space for love.

278

I urge all communities to look to San Francisco and to look at the experience that is going on here and the support system that has been formed here. . . . Communities [all over the country] should look toward this community as a model and learn from it and set up systems like it. . . . We are going to need them. It's strange, so many of the people that I have worked with have come to a point where they have honestly said, "You know, Irene, I don't want to live without AIDS. I don't want to live the way I lived before because there was no love and support involved."

I worked with one person who was really quite healthy and radiant, and he had been seeking out all different forms of healing. He was doing psychic healing, colon cleansing, microbiotic diets. He really leaned toward his psychic healing, but he was doing body work, meditation and yoga, and he just went from one form of healing to another. And I remember one day in yoga class, I asked him, "Chris, why do you continually search for more and more healing? Can you not sit down and acknowledge the healing that you have received?" He replied that he could, but what had happened was that he had reached the point of needing more and more healing; the same pattern we get into in living: never sitting down and acknowledging what we have, but continuing a search when there is really no need for one.

Chris told me at that point that he was really afraid of dying but that he was also very afraid of living without AIDS because it was with AIDS that he had found so much love, support, and caring. It was AIDS that opened this entire path of growth for him. He talked about AIDS being an opportunity for growth. I know that a lot of people with AIDS [are tired of hearing people] say that it's an opportunity, and sometimes it is kind of hard to see it, but it is true. It's an opportunity for those people with AIDS to grow and finish their business, to explore the flowers and the trees, and to open, receive, and give love. It's an enormous opportunity for growth, and it's also an enormous opportunity for growth for those people who form the support system.

The people who have AIDS have contracted a disease that no one seems to know anything about. They have a disease where there's an enormous amount of fear not only from their neighbors, but also from most of . . . society. . . . They're faced with a disease that the medical community [really knows nothing] about, and, therefore, the medical treatments are coming from research and experimentation. All of the treatment that is given for AIDS at this point is for the opportunistic infection that has set in. Granted some of these treatments can, for a short period of time, help arrest the infection, but what these treatments do, in turn, is knock one's immune system down further, and the immune system is where the disease lies. So actually, at this point, one is kind of in a catch-22. One can either not have treatment, or one can have medical treatment that knocks the immune system further down. So this is quite a challenge in itself—what to do?

As I said earlier, one is also faced with a society that has an enormous amount of fear of the disease. One is also faced with rejection and a total lack of understanding as to what is going on. One is caught in a corner, and not only that, but from the day you are diagnosed, you are told that you have x amount of time to live, even though people do not know anything about the disease. You are sort of doomed by society to die from the first day of diagnosis. [While we have an enormous amount of support] in the

San Francisco Bay area for those people with AIDS, the support [really] exists to help the people with AIDS die. From the day you are diagnosed, you are told how to make out your will, and you are told that there are counselors available to help you do these things. That's wonderful; you need to handle the practical side of living. However, no one ever comes to you and tells you that there isn't really anything known about the disease and maybe you will live.

And that, maybe, you can heal yourself! To this day, there still isn't an organization formed for alternative therapies, and from all of the information that I've heard, or that I've read, people who are doing alternative medicine are doing well. A lot of them are doing well, and granted, there are people who are dying on alternatives just as much as they are dying with, and without, regular medical treatment, but it seems that the quality of life is much higher with people doing alternative therapies; there needs to be a movement for alternatives for people with AIDS, just like cancer patients.

So you have an enormous challenge there. You have the challenge of really getting out there if you have AIDS and seeking knowledge and information on therapies that are helping people get better. This is something that is not made available easily; it is something that you really have to search for. Another challenge of AIDS, if you are a member of a gay community, is that you are possibly faced with people who are constantly dying around you. I think that the main challenge, at this time, is that there just is not enough funding. Funding just has not come out into the realm of research or in the realm of information for people with AIDS. There are loaded hospitals; there are health-care organizations that cannot even find the funding to stay alive, much less offer the care that is needed for a group of people who reach the level of illness that they reach with AIDS. What I believe is happening, especially in our health-care profession, is that up until this time, people, groups of people who become extremely ill and die in any large numbers have been our senior citizens, and the health-care profession really isn't prepared to care for relatively young people who reach this level of debilitation and keep on living.

Here we have a group of people in their twenties and thirties who may not have paid any Social Security. They may not have worked for an organization that took taxes out of their paychecks. There is nothing to fall back on. They don't have life savings. They don't have insurance policies. They don't have hospitalization insurance. There is a whole group of people who need to be cared for who have not had thirty, forty, or fifty years to plan for it, and the funding just is not coming in. I do not know what is going to be done when more people come down with AIDS. Who is going to care for these people? We must have funding and we must have volunteers.

Chapter 10

AIDS **in Prison**

In contrast to the patients who are taken care of by wonderful support systems, AIDS patients who are incarcerated in our prisons have no support whatsoever. They are kept in isolated rooms for months and months. They have virtually no contact with other inmates, are never able to go outside into the fresh air and sunshine, and have no chance to exercise their already weak physical bodies. Without the use of a radio or TV they sit all day long in their small cells, isolated and unattended; they receive no special care and they have no chance to talk about the deplorable condition they are in.

I made dozens of telephone calls to Washington, and I talked to every conceivable source who had anything to do with the prison system. I was told that they had "no problems whatsoever with any inmates who had AIDS." In fact, they told me they knew of only four AIDS patients— and these had been released. All the others had supposedly died prior to incarceration!

Twenty-four hours later, I was on a plane to California to see for myself. Do AIDS patients in correctional institutions get adequate care? In one prison alone, there were eight young men with AIDS. Each one was in his own isolated cell; each one was deprived of outdoor exercise or other sports activities that they were still able to perform. They were in an utter state of depression and despair without a chance for any improvement. The food was so untenable that half of them were unable to swallow because of their mouth and throat infections. And what services were available only slowed down even more if they complained.

One man who was virtually covered with Kaposi's sarcoma begged to be given permission to have some radiation treatment and never received an answer. Every day he watched the spread of his disease and every day he hoped—in vain—for a doctor's visit and the news that he was accepted for radiation. I had a lengthy discussion with the prison physician and it soon became very clear that he knew very little about AIDS and was really not that interested. He had had a county practice previously, and when he retired he moved to California, where he was offered this prison position. I asked him, as a personal favor, to arrange for radiation treatment for this man and promised to make all the necessary arrangements if that would help any. He casually said, "Well, one of these days, we will probably send him to San Francisco for a treatment." I told him that this man needed more than one treatment and that San Francisco General could easily house him and take care of his needs.

Another physician, at the same prison, talked about a different inmate who had AIDS but claimed not to be homosexual. It was clear that this doctor did not believe

284

any of his patients, and that anyone with AIDS was categorically homosexual. I could get nowhere with him. He was very judgmental and also poorly informed about the nature of AIDS. I reassured him that many blood transfusion patients and IV drug users also showed AIDS, and that this prisoner had a history of an earlier blood transfusion that could easily have been the source of his infection. But, obviously, this doctor did not want to be bothered with this inmate or with what I was saying. It fell on deaf ears.

With a staff of so-called care-givers who are so negative, clearly vindictive, and out for revenge, it is no surprise that prison is the worst place to be if you have AIDS.

One of the inmates was really desperate. He begged me to talk to the people in charge. His family did not know that he was in prison; they did not know that he was homosexual; they did not know that he was dying of AIDS. He urgently needed to talk to someone before he went crazy. He had neither radio nor TV. Books were not available to him; he suspected the authorities did not want to send books to the infirmary because they did not want to "spread AIDS" throughout the prison.

Three weeks earlier he had sent a written request to talk to the counselor, and the day before my visit he had received a reply that said, "State your concern"; no appointment, no set time!

He felt his death was imminent, and he wanted to put his house in order and leave a letter to his family, but had no one who was interested in his needs.

I talked again to the prisoner who insisted he had gotten AIDS from a transfusion—he also insisted that he was innocent of any crime. He did not want to die in jail. He desperately wanted to explore all possible treatment

285

chances he had on the outside and painted a truly horrible picture of the prison system in America. I was thinking of Amnesty International, of which I am a proud member, and the thought occurred to me that it is high time we took a look at the prison system in our own country, and that we learn to treat our fellow human beings with more compassion and humanity, with intelligence and much less vindictiveness.

In the late summer or early fall of 1985, the first reports about AIDS in prisons began to appear in the news media: "AIDS Not Yet a Major Problem in State Prison." In the Harrisonburg *Daily News Record* of August 13, 1985: "AIDS in Prison May Cause State Problems." An article in a Richmond, Virginia, paper stated: "AIDS in Virginia Prisons is lower than in states like New York, but is higher than the national average, and is a matter of great concern." Edward Murray, the corrections director who made that statement, went on to say, "We hope it does not get out of hand."

A study sponsored by the National Institute of Justice and the American Correctional Association found 179 AIDS cases in prisons in the United States, with three quarters coming from New York, New Jersey, and Pennsylvania facilities. Another 11 percent are in the South Atlantic region, which includes Maryland, Virginia, West Virginia, the District of Columbia, the Carolinas, Georgia, and Florida.

The five cases that were in Virginia at the time (which has a total inmate population of 10,800) compares to a total of about a hundred cases reported among the state's 5.5 million inhabitants since 1982.

Dr. Robert Frey, the head physician of the national

prison system, said that inmates with AIDS are, or were, mostly intravenous drug users or homosexuals. He said there is no way of telling how they got the disease or whether they contracted it in prison. The correctional department has issued pamphlets to inmates and staff to both calm and inform them. Everybody is concerned about it. Frey said, "Legal problems could arise from the department's policy to isolate AIDS prisoners, or from a change of that policy. The fellow we now have with AIDS strongly resents his isolation. He considers it punitive and says he might as well be dead." Frey said his office established the isolation policy to keep the disease from spreading to others. "It is pretty restrictive and I understand why a prisoner would be upset about it," he said. "But if we wouldn't isolate, I'm certain the other prisoners would strenuously object. They have had problems with this in other state systems and I understand one AIDS victim was even murdered."

Frey also said that "AIDS patients are shunned by other prisoners and as much as possible by corrections officers!" Chan Kendrick, executive director of the American Civil Liberties Union of Virginia, said that "he hasn't received a single letter or call of complaint about the isolation procedure."

It seems to me that it is the other way around: The inmates should be isolated to protect *the patient,* not the other inmates, from infections. Dr. Frey states that the isolation procedure was instigated to prevent the spread of AIDS within the prison system. But this is the wrong reason for starting such a restrictive policy. An AIDS patient's immune system is so reduced, that the slightest infection, or cold from another inmate, can be a death penalty.

Corrections officers in New York State went to court

to try to avoid having contact with AIDS inmates, but they lost their case. Since prisoners are not routinely tested for AIDS when they enter the system, anyone can be a carrier, and until they get sick and are then transferred to a medical facility, no one will ever know.

A newspaper report from Valhalla, New York, shed light on some of the problems that cause concern in the correctional institutions: "A Westchester county jail inmate stricken with AIDS harassed other people by spitting on them." The same inmate, charged with stealing property and committing felonies, was allowed to plead guilty to a misdemeanor and released, partly because he had AIDS. He was not required to appear in court because court officers balked at handling him. In Minnesota, inmates at the Stillwater prison were locked in their cells after one of their number was diagnosed with AIDS-related complex, a milder form of the disease, which might, however, lead to AIDS. Hundreds of other inmates had planned to demonstrate and demand to be tested for AIDS, and a guard who refused to search prisoners was suspended. Prison officials said they would educate prisoners and staff during the two-week lockup.

In prisons around the nation, AIDS is causing unrest, confusion, and fear. A 1985 survey of state and federal prison systems by the Associated Press found widely varying policies for dealing with prisoners with AIDS, and in some cases no policies at all. According to the survey, since 1981, several hundred cases of AIDS have been reported and confirmed in prisons, most of them in the Northeast.

There have been thirty confirmed cases in the federal system's forty-six prisons. Since routine testing of inmates is not done, it is impossible to say how widespread the deadly disease is in our prisons. Misinformation and fear abound, however. In Delaware, guards began to wear rubber gloves when transporting inmates who they said were "known homosexuals"—they were ordered to stop wearing gloves unless the prisoner was known to have a communicable disease. In Arizona, three guards were granted transfers from the state prison in Florence after an AIDS case was confirmed. "We feel that homosexual contact in prisons is rampant," said Margaret Hoyos, a spokeswoman for the guard's union. "The Department of Corrections is a little too conservative in its estimate of how AIDS is transmitted." She said officers walking through the prison yards are often pelted with feces and urine. Although, in most correctional institutions, prisoners are isolated and segregated, officers don't seem to be protected enough.

In Michigan, the policy calls for AIDS victims to remain in the general prison population unless they are physically ill. Routine testing for AIDS is generally rejected by prison officials as unnecessary, although the initial test only verifies if a person has been exposed to the virus thought to cause AIDS.

It has become more than evident to me that, for all our advances, there is still a horrible bias against homosexuals. There is tremendous fear of a still incurable disease. As of this writing, there have been no effective attempts to keep the prison population calm. The complete lack of coordinated regulations and policy have already started to create a panic about the spread of this epidemic in a penal system that itself fosters drug use and homosexuality. The refusal to make condoms available to inmates is clearly a form of denial: Any ex-convict can confirm the large degree of sexual activity in our prisons.

The grimmest part of all of this is the ignorance of AIDS in general and the absolute lack of understanding, love, and compassion for those who are terminally ill and receive no treatment.

I cannot imagine where we would be without the help of wonderful new volunteers, all former participants of our workshops. Many of them have taken on the task of visiting sick inmates, supplying them with TV, trying to help shorten their long days in isolation. More important, these volunteers create human contact. They are nonjudgmental, not punitive, and they understand the prisoner's plight.

On one occasion in California's Vacaville prison, an evening was organized where every inmate with AIDS was allowed to have two visitors. Except for our own volunteers, only two people showed up—it was a sad revelation of their extreme isolation from and rejection by family and society.

A fifty-four-year-old man wrote "Dear Abby" the following letter:

> I am just beginning to serve a fifty-year prison sentence. There is absolutely no chance of my being released earlier, hence I am resigned to the fate of having to die in prison. Why must I be compelled to go on suffering the dehumanization of prison confinement until I die? Is there any way I can volunteer to be a guinea pig to advance medical science in its search for a cure of AIDS or cancer? Although I am not a homosexual, I do not hate my fellow human beings for being human. Any assistance you can render in this matter would be greatly appreciated. Perhaps by death, I will be able to accomplish that which

I failed so miserably to do in my 54 years of life. Thank you.

No. 15621-008

It makes me sad to read these lines. How much such people could contribute to society instead of being locked up in a system that is by its very nature punitive and dehumanizing—a system which locks up thousands of relatively young and strong people and lets them sit and vegetate, killing the hours, the days, and the years at the taxpayers' expense.

I started a prison project on the Island of Maui years before the onset of AIDS. I came in contact with people from all over the world, including men and women who were potential mass murderers, who had committed violent crimes. They were often perpetrators of abuse, violence, and incest. Many of these people came to my workshops, which are always held in confidential and caring environments. I have found that with nonpunitive and nonjudgmental people listening to them, these men and women were able to be healed *before* they committed a crime. If it is possible to do that with one hundred people in five days, then we should be able to organize in our prisons an approach that makes use of the inmates' time in a healing, constructive way.

If indeed they could be healed of their early traumas and negative conditioning, then prisoners would be ready for release in a much better, healthier, and less destructive frame of mind. We did that in the prison on Maui with our first pilot project and we are very proud of the institution, which was generous enough to give us and its inmates a chance.

291

* * *

I conducted several interviews with young prisoners with AIDS *during my trip to California. The first interview, which follows, was with the inmate who so badly needed treatment for his Kaposi's sarcoma.*

PATIENT: Look at my right foot here. It is very painful, you know, and it started in just one toe and they kept saying it was a fungus.

ELISABETH: *That was in the county jail?*

PATIENT: Yes, and they were giving me ointments and creams. They never bothered to really test me to see what it was, and then I got to this place and they told me that I would see the foot doctor and he was giving me different types of antibiotics, and nothing seemed to help; then I saw this breaking out on my leg, and I said, "Doctor, that's the same thing that's on my toe," and he says, "Oh, it's just varicose veins, don't worry about it," and it started getting worse. I showed it to him again, and he sent me to see another doctor, and he biopsied the one spot that broke out on my arm; then two weeks later he biopsied a spot on my leg, and they both came back, "not AIDS." Then he sent them to the naval hospital and they came back, "Kaposi's sarcoma." And then they knew where we were. By that time the spots were advancing on both legs, and since then, I've been trying to get an 1170, which is to release me so that I can go get medical help. They won't do it. I can't get anybody around here to cooperate. No one wants to take the responsibility in here. It's like, they say, "You aren't terminal yet." In other words, they want to make sure I'm dead before they release me. It's the most ridiculous thing I've ever heard. In other words, "We are going to kill you before we release you."

ELISABETH: *How long are you in for?*

PATIENT: I've got two and a half years to go, but I'll never live to see my release date. This just happened since January and in six months' time, look at it. I've got it advancing up here. I've got it now breaking out on my chest, and I'm still trying to get help.

ELISABETH: *I will talk to your doctor.*

PATIENT: Finally, they sent me to San Francisco and a doctor looked at me and he said, "There's lots of things we can do to him. We can give him radiation treatment; chemotherapy." The red tape they've got around here is, like I'm going to be dead by the time they ever get me treated, and so I've got to try and get out of here—get an early parole date—because isn't my right to life more than their right to punish me? I'm not here for any violence.

ELISABETH: *What are you in for?*

PATIENT: I'm here for a robbery which I didn't commit, and I'm still appealing it. I pleaded "no contest" because they refused to let me have a private lawyer, and the guy they are looking for is six feet two inches with blond hair and blond mustache, and they got me down as that person and that's why I'm here, and because of that, they're going to end up killing me. I'm so mad, I can't see straight. I would have already gotten treatment if I were on the street, but because

I'm here, it's already gotten this bad. And it's probably going to get much worse before I get any help. I'm very angry and upset.

ELISABETH: *I don't blame you.*

PATIENT: I'm so happy that you're here. It's the best thing that's happened to me.

ELISABETH: *You see, that's really our role, to get help early for everybody.*

PATIENT: Isn't the right to life more important than punishment, making sure we have our punishment—especially for something we didn't do. If we try and tell the System that, it's impossible, no one believes you. It's like everybody claims to be innocent, and they're not; but I happen to be innocent. I've been screaming for six months. I've been trying to see my counselor, to get help, for two months and he completely ignores my letters and won't see me. I sent one request on the sixth to him. I sent several before that. And, on the twenty-fifth, he sent this back here, "What is it you want? State your problem and return." He's just being a complete asshole. See right here, "I keep filling out these slips to see you, you don't reply." And he has to, initially, want to get an 1170 to get me out of here. He's a C.C. number two [*counselor*]. He refuses to see me, probably because of the AIDS. I'm so mad. It's so painful. There are times I can't get out of bed. See that cup right there? I have to pee in that cup sometimes and just throw it out the window because I can't get out of bed to even go to the toilet, it's so painful. It's ridiculous. Here's where it started, right here [*looks at toes*]. I've seen other people with toes like that, and they probably don't know what it is—it's probably AIDS, an early diagnosis and they don't recognize it.

ELISABETH: *And that's the most painful part?*

PATIENT: That's the painful part. I keep telling the doctors, "Look it's advancing over my whole body, can't you get me help?" And you know how the red tape is. Now I'm getting them up here on my chest and my mouth is starting to get sore, they're still not doing anything for me. Right now, this is my morning medicine. All these are vitamin pills. This is antifungus for my toes. That's the extent of my medication right there, other than some pain pills I have. Until you're dying, we can't release you. At least the other doctors are willing to cooperate with an 1170, but [this one] says that this isn't true, and he doesn't know that this is terminal. He figures it is not terminal until you can't get out of bed, can't move, and then you're terminal. In other words, we want to be sure you can't be cured before we release you, and that's the most ridiculous thing I've ever heard.

ELISABETH: *Were you shocked when the diagnosis was* AIDS?

PATIENT: They verified my diagnosis of AIDS in March. I, more or less, knew what I had. I can't get these doctors around here to do anything. And it's so frustrating, to know that you need help and you can't have it. Who helped me the most? None of them.

ELISABETH: *Do you have any outside moral support?*

PATIENT: No. I have one friend who came to see me and he was going to see my judge for me. Three days later, he died. My best friend, he died from something, I don't know. I just called home and I found out he died three days after his visit, and there went all my help out the window. It's changed my life considerably, basically due to the fact that I'm now forty-two. My life was getting stable. My friends are old and established. My life was just getting comfortable and now for this to happen, and to have it change at this point, because I love old age and I've always dreamed of being old myself, because I look forward to my older, retirement years.

ELISABETH: *What kind of work did you do?*

PATIENT: Well, I used to own a nightclub and I've always been in business for myself. I've been in trouble with the law for the past ten years, not really major stuff, but minor problems, and it was with drugs, which was stupidity on my part. Now that I'm older, I can see that I've got my life ahead of me and I want to straighten it out. To know that I'm being cheated out of it— I'm very upset. I would like to go see my family before I die, and to be locked up and kept away from that opportunity, to know that I may die in here, and that my mother hasn't seen me in fifteen years and may be cheated out of that last visit from me, and me to her.

ELISABETH: *Where do they live?*

PATIENT: She lives in Florida.

ELISABETH: *Can I write to you when I leave?*

PATIENT: Yes, I would like that.

ELISABETH: *I will write to you. You haven't seen your mother in fifteen years? Can I write to her?*

PATIENT: I would, but I don't want to worry her, knowing I'm in prison, and stuff— I'd just like to go and see her. My family would like to see me. I'd like to see them very much. There's no way I can until I get out of here. It's very frustrating to know that.

ELISABETH: *So they don't know?*

PATIENT: No.

ELISABETH: [*Asks the physician who has arrived*] *Is it possible that he can get some irradiation treatment?*

DOCTOR: Oh yes, oh yes. The problem is his getting aligned to the areas around here. There are two places between here and San Francisco that do it. Down in San Francisco, where he went, should have called us back a long time ago.

PATIENT: I mentioned to her about the 1170 that I had been trying to get it. You said I'm not terminal.

DOCTOR: Yes, the only way we can give the 1170 is in the case of imminent death.

PATIENT: But it's also a release for medical reasons when you are terminal if you don't get released, and that is the case here.

ELISABETH: *Do you feel that you get enough medical care here?*

PATIENT: No.

ELISABETH: *It's not the same as outside?*

PATIENT: No, it's not.

ELISABETH: *Are you expecting to be paroled?*

PATIENT: I'm supposed to be paroled, I think, November 10, 1986.

ELISABETH: *That's very soon. It's in November.*

PATIENT: Oh, but that doesn't matter.

ELISABETH: *Yes, but it's still better than five years from now. Right?*

PATIENT: I have no push button for emergency calls. They would have to move me from this room to another room or the ICU. That's the recommendation that I have heard. A person very intensely ill, to watch him twenty-four hours in ICU. But I would still rather— They send you to the general hospital anyway, so I would rather, you know, be in San Francisco General. Put fifty, sixty locks and chains on my feet, I don't care. This is the first time I've ever been in prison.

ELISABETH: *What did you say you were in for?*

PATIENT: I'm in for burglary . . . to support my drug habit. This is why I have this immune deficiency.

ELISABETH: *From the injections?*

PATIENT: Yes.

ELISABETH: *Does your family know about your* AIDS?

PATIENT: No. If you're asking me if they know, they don't know that I'm dying—no.

ELISABETH: *You don't have a support system from there?*

PATIENT: I have nothing coming in, nothing going out. No letters, no friends. I have no support at all. Nothing at all.

ELISABETH: *You have no girlfriend? No support system? Nothing?*

PATIENT: I have nobody to write to—I have nobody. I've tried in some kind of way that AIDS patients that are out could write to me if they feel they're up to it.

ELISABETH: *Do you want to correspond with one?*

PATIENT: Yes! That's what I would like. They think they're too good for me because I'm in prison this one time.

ELISABETH: *I will tell some of my patients to write to you. Write down your address, please.*

PATIENT: I'll give you the name and how they can reach everybody here. And that will be for anybody you talk to. You want my prison number?

ELISABETH: *Yes. Can you give me your official address? I have so many AIDS patients who would love to help somebody else with the same problem. You're helping each other, you know. How do you see the future?*

PATIENT: How do I see the future? To live in happiness is the only thing that will content my soul before I leave.

ELISABETH: *There's a marvelous support system among AIDS patients in this whole area.*

PATIENT: If I had an 1170, I guarantee you I would be there. I will be there. I went through it already. I know I'm the patient. I went through the symptoms. There are things that are personal in a human organism.

299

ELISABETH: *That the patient knows from his own experience.*

PATIENT: One thing: I need to have a telephone directory of New York State . . . three places. Maybe I could take care of that with the sergeant. I need a directory for New York State, for Florida, and for Puerto Rico.

ELISABETH: *Get back in touch with your family. Your sergeant can help you.*

PATIENT: I hope so. I haven't spoken to him about it.

ELISABETH: *Talk to him. How can we help you the most?*

PATIENT: My friend, if there's any charity, a collection, or whatever, they can send me packages weighing thirty pounds. There's such things that I don't eat. I went down, when I was being screened, to seventy pounds. I have anorexia—I have loss of appetite—the only thing I love to eat is Top Ramen Chinese noodles, beef flavor.

ELISABETH: *Yes, I know them well.*

PATIENT: They cost twenty-five cents apiece. And I'm talking about the same person that's going to write to me! I spend three, four, five days, sometimes a whole week, without eating anything. I try and I just spit it out because it's not what I want. My mouth is too delicate for chewing, and those noodles, they help me. The nice beef broth is enriching. It has all the vitamins.

ELISABETH: *What are your greatest needs now?*

PATIENT: I have no lawyer. I want to get an 1170. This is my first time ever in prison.

ELISABETH: *Talk to the MAC Committee and they can arrange something for you. The MAC Committee is made up of inmates and they have a couple of attorneys who will help you do what you're trying to do.*

PATIENT: I'm not giving up. I'm fighting, but the sooner I can get a friend, the better I'll be.

The following interview was with an AIDS patient who had been married and had a six-year-old son. The prison refused to give him medical treatment:

ELISABETH: *How long have you been here?*

PATIENT: Two months.

ELISABETH: *Two months. And how long are you in for?*

PATIENT: Two years, eight months.

ELISABETH: *That's rough. Did you know you had this medical problem before you came in?*

PATIENT: Yes. I went in front of the judge, and I was already diagnosed, and he gave me six years anyway.

ELISABETH: *How can people do that to each other? What are you in for?*

PATIENT: Somebody did the burglary and I got the goods and I was selling it, so they pinned it on me.

ELISABETH: *Did you get any treatment before you came in?*

PATIENT: No.

ELISABETH: *I'm a physician and I am trying to get all the information so that we can help everybody inside*

301

and outside the penal system. But you need to tell me what I can do to help inmates with AIDS.

PATIENT: Get them out of a place like this. All they were giving me was something for my nerves—Valium—keep 'em calm, keep 'em calm, keep 'em calm. They told me straight out, "You're going to die."

ELISABETH: *Which is not necessarily true, you know that.*

PATIENT: I'm scared, and they come out and tell me something like that. I go in front of the judge— I had an appointment to go to San Francisco General Hospital, to see the psychiatrist, and the judge overlooked all that and sentenced me here. I didn't kill nobody. To me, it's like it's Death Row right here.

ELISABETH: *Do you have a support system outside?*

PATIENT: My mom and dad. I'm divorced, and I've got a six-year-old son. They write me and see how I'm doing.

ELISABETH: *Your mom and dad know what's medically wrong?*

PATIENT: Yes.

ELISABETH: *And they support you?*

PATIENT: Yes.

ELISABETH: *Boy, are you lucky! At least you have that.*

PATIENT: Well, my dad's going to the doctor, too, because he's pretty sick. He's had cancer. It's hard for my mom to deal with both.

ELISABETH: *Where do they live?*

PATIENT: In Monterey County. I didn't want none of this to be on the news at first, and they brought it all on the news—the way the county jail there treated me. They wear masks and gloves. They treat you like you're an animal in a cage and throw peanuts at you.

ELISABETH: *But not here?*

PATIENT: Some of them treat you normally. You've got the ones that still don't want anything to do with you. If you were to fall on the floor, they're not going to come up to you and give you mouth-to-mouth.

ELISABETH: *How can we help you?*

PATIENT: Well, I've got an 1170 that's got to be back in court. The judge granted it. It takes a couple of years off my sentence. I think I was sent to prison because of my disease; they didn't want me in that county, because you don't ever hear of it in Monterey County, I guess, and they didn't want me around there.

The following vignettes are taken from three terribly moving case histories with three other inmates with AIDS:

This young man, Z. L., believed that he was in the wrong place at the wrong time. He was picked up by the police during a shuffling of people when a policeman was roughing up a man who was in an argument after a minor car accident. The policeman tried to handcuff the young driver and Z. L. went to his rescue as he knew that the handcuffed man was innocent. It was to no avail. He was taken to jail.

He asked to call a lawyer or a friend. He believed that he was entitled to at least one phone call. But it was denied. After a night of trying to get some sleep on the floor of the jail, some other "overnight guests" attacked him and abused him. He was afraid for his life but the guards ignored his screams for help. A sadistic grin on the face of one of the guards made Z. L. believe that he actually got some sadistic pleasure listening to the sounds of the assault.

When he was discharged, Z. L. was shaken up and tried to keep to himself. It was only two and a half years later that he shared this trauma during one of our workshops, where he was able to ventilate his rage, his feelings of impotence and helplessness. It was the memory of this man that first led me to think about jails and prisons, and eventually, to go and see for myself, to find out what the conditions are in places that perpetuate so much cruelty. I also wanted to see for myself how AIDS patients were treated.

But I found no healers, no helpers, no caring physicians to attend to the AIDS patients. And where were the ministers who preach about love from their pulpits?

Z. L. has since died of AIDS. He was only twenty-four years old. Shortly before he died, he said to me, "I have just started to live. I had a lovely girlfriend and planned to go into social work. I loved to help people in need! Why is this happening to me?"

Z. L. lost his sight before he died and one of the few hobbies he had enjoyed was painting. He wistfully said, "I think this is the nastiest disease that ever hit this planet Earth. You recuperate from your terrible diarrhea only to have trouble breathing, and when you learn to gasp for your every breath and finally recuperate a little from that, then it affects your brain or you become blind." The night before he died, he welcomed death as an end to his suffering and, hopefully, a new beginning.

R. C., a thirty-two-year-old inmate, dates the onset of symptoms to April 1984 with a verification of AIDS more than a year later, in June 1985. His first reaction was surprise, followed by a deep apprehension and then anger that "nothing was done medically to detect this earlier while I was in the county jail."

Since then he went through a tremendous sense of loneliness and deep depression, "knowing that one day soon life will end and those left behind will suffer grief." He feels that his life has not changed all that much except for the fact that he is aware that "I may die within a few years" and "my 'I don't care anymore' attitude has surfaced."

People who helped him financially and supported him, prior to his illness, have stopped all support. He, too, like so many of the inmates, asked for a TV and pen pals in order not to feel so desperately lonely. Asked about other friends, he makes it clear that everyone has deserted him and shunned him; his only pal is a fellow AIDS patient.

Asked about the response of his family, he sadly and thoughtfully responded: "I don't really know yet. But I expect that they will be confused and not understand. They will be angry also as they don't understand or care to believe that I am gay."

He looks at the future with great uncertainty and feels very concerned—"being alone doesn't help either." When asked how we could help, his answer reflected almost all the answers we received by inmates: "By seeing that my medical needs are not neglected, and that I be allowed to die among my own kind: gay men with AIDS in a real licensed hospital!" He also asked for something to keep his mind busy, reading material—anything to occupy him—"I am locked up in this room twenty-four hours a day with nothing to do but look out of my window."

Since most inmates with AIDS were locked up all day and night, they had few distractions from their own thoughts, grief, and physical and emotional anguish. Counselors did not want to get near them, literature was withheld ("They are afraid others may catch the disease by reading the same books"). Only a few privileged (and financially better off) prisoners had either radio or TV. Most of them had none or very few visitors. They all were eager for a pen pal.

J. R. is a twenty-nine-year-old Monterey, California, man who showed the first symptoms of his disease in June 1984. The diagnosis of AIDS was verified the following January, and he reacted to it with a tremendous amount of "scariness." He feels that he never knows if he is going to wake up the following morning and is totally aware that this disease is a death sentence.

Asked about the future, he says: "I hope that they find a cure and that I am out of here [prison] to see the future. My greatest need is to be with my family for what time

I have left." At the time of my visiting him in prison, he stated that "I am scared, but little by little I am learning to deal with my illness."

His greatest wishes were to have a TV and a pen pal so he would not feel so isolated in spite of the fact that he was in isolation in his correctional institution; he did not expect this to change as long as he was incarcerated.

October 22, 1985

Dear Elisabeth,

Hi. I certainly hope that these few words will find you well, and thank God that you weren't lynched for trying or desiring to build a center for poor innocent AIDS victim children on your own land. That really hurt me to my heart. It's so sad. Oh! I found out that the money you had sent to your secretary in San Francisco to get me a TV, that accidentally they bought someone else one with it. At first I felt hurt when everyone else who you interviewed got TVs, and people would tell me, I think you got left out because you were black. "Where is your TV? You're the only one who didn't get one." Then when I wrote you and you told me on September 10 that you had forwarded money to San Francisco to your secretary in an attempt to expedite me getting one, then I found out that they accidentally spent the money to buy someone else one with the money that was for mine. But that is okay. One of the ladies from the foundation, who explained the mistake to me in a letter, said that she would buy me one out of her own money, even though it would place a strain on her. I wrote her back and said that I did not

307

want her to do that, because I could not enjoy it, knowing that she or possibly her children, etc., went without to buy me a TV. One of these days I will get one. But you left a lasting impression on me when you visited me in the prison hospital. Afterwards, I said Elisabeth is such a remarkable woman, always giving of herself to help the less fortunate. Sometimes I really feel that people miss the real essence of life, because they feel that is about all that you can receive, so wrong they are, for I have learned even under these circumstances and through these trying times, that sometimes, so often you get so much more by giving than by receiving. I'm not talking about materialistic gain, I'm speaking about mental and spiritual gain. For so long such things were of no value to me. Now, as I sit around here having been diagnosed as having crossed over the line from ARC to AIDS, it makes one realize how beautiful life is. Of course, there are times when I feel so depressed that I do not believe no language has the appropriate words to express adequately how depressed I feel. I think about the things I've done; I think about the things I've desired to do; I think about how I used to make plans like in 1981 I said the Olympics are going to be in Los Angeles, California. I am going to go. I am a realistic person. I don't make any long-range plans, for I have come to the conclusion, it's not the longevity that makes one's life either one that was worthy of living or one that was un-worthy, it's the quality that makes life worth it. I've found in my life as in so many others' lives the old saying "Into Each Life Some Rain Must Fall," but that's okay. because I now see and realize that it is so true, that as rain falls into each life, my new saying, and I believe it is, "Into Each Life Some Sun Must Shine." Sometimes we got to open the door to let it in. Me, I desire to bring if but a small sparkle of sun to someone's life, let it be, for then I will know that my life has not been in vain. Yes, Elisabeth, you can print my poems, any that you wish in your quarterly, as long as you promise to send me a copy. Just maybe some of them will slide through the shade of someone's life, and in its place bring a little sparkle of sun. I can not give you the copyright for I am seriously considering gathering a number of my poems and assembling a book of them. As I said I am not sure yet, but I really want to, for deep inside I feel that just maybe God has given me the potential to bring a ray of sun to some otherwise sunless life through my writings. As I say I must really consider, for the clock is constantly running. Time waits upon no being. Give me your opinion. A lot of us are no longer in the hospital, but we are cramped up in this little hole in the wall. Yet it brings you closer to people. For you can be realistic and say I'm scared for I know not if I have very many more to-morrows, yet me personally I believe in the Supreme Being, and that alone with faith and confidence in one's self, as well as the will, can do what nothing else can even come close to doing. Yes, I must still take medicine for my head pains, for they get terrible at times. Yet I know all things have a purpose. Though I am not exactly pleased as to the circumstances we met under, I believe our meeting was meant to be. I do not know if you realize it, but there are times when just the thought of you brings sunshine in my life to a day that would otherwise not have any. Like today, I wonder if the sun shined; I wonder if it rained. Really, I do not know, but something about the thought of you brought me sunshine and I thank you. I shall close this letter, but my admiration, respect, love and appreciation of you entering my life shall remain always, even throughout eternity, and when eternity ceases to be no more, my respect, thankfulness, appreciation for the sun that you brought into my life without you even knowing it shall remain as strong then as it is now, if not stronger.

Love always,
Larry

The following letter from Nancy Jaicks and Robert Alexander, my assistants on the West Coast, brings us up to date on conditions in the prisons I visited.

August 24, 1987

Dear Elisabeth,

Your recollection of prisoners with AIDS at the California Medical Facility is based on conditions in August 1985. You have asked for an update. It is based on our observations since then until August 1987. Conditions will continue to change, hopefully for the better.

When prisoners diagnosed seropositive were first detected in the prison population, a decision was made by the director of the Department of Corrections to segregate them in one facility in the state.

310

This was said to be for protection of such prisoners from violent attacks by other inmates. This reason may have been valid at the time or it could have reflected the paranoia of the administration itself.

Since November 3, 1986, when we started to visit the AIDS wing, we have yet to find an inmate who is afraid of being released to the general prison population because of his stigma. Some need protective custody for other reasons. When we have walked down a long corridor with a group of AIDS wing inmates, we have heard them greet their friends or acquaintances cordially with no signs of animosity.

The first eight or ten seropositive prisoners were housed in a small dormitory containing ten double-tiered cots. Sanitary facilities were minimal and privacy was nonexistent. After the numbers reached twenty, they were moved into a separated wing containing about forty cells. The single cells soon became double-occupancy "houses." When inmates became ill with an "opportunistic disease," they were transferred to the prison hospital.

When the population of the AIDS wing reached eighty, an adjacent wing was added and the present population is about 115. Each wing has a TV room. Between the two wings is a room which has been equipped with fixed tables and stools as a cafeteria. The evening meal is now served hot from a steam table. This is a dramatic improvement.

Only one small exercise yard is available to both wings. For some reason the inmates of the two wings are separated from each other. They use the yard alternately. They also have alternate use of the cafeteria for card playing. They have access to the gymnasium when it is not in use by the "Main Line."

A doctor visits each wing once a week. Medicine prescribed is dispensed by MTAs every day from a room on one of the wings. Inmates dread going to the hospital, which is under court order to become accredited by the end of next year. Conditions of AIDS patients' care in the hospital are the worst we can imagine. Some medical personnel are judgmental and completely devoid of sympathy or understanding.

One AIDS wing contains a cell designated "Law Library." It is a sham containing only case-law records. Each wing contains a cell devoted to consultation with a psychologist or counselor. Lessons in art and writing have been started and quickly terminated for reasons we do not know. Our visits have been consistent once a week since November 3, 1986. We fill a token need for support- or rap-group leadership.

A start has been made in AIDS education. Staff directly involved in the AIDS wings has attended a two-day workshop outside and a day-long workshop in-house. They have volunteered to work in the AIDS wings. Their response to inmates appears to reflect genuine understanding of the disease and the inmate's plight.

Inmates of the AIDS wings appear to have as much AIDS education as anyone, but are always eager for more. As far as we know this is all self-acquired. They seek information desperately on when to turn for help when released.

Education of prison staff at Vacaville is focused

on self-protection in case of bloody incident. They are appropriately taught to assume that every prisoner has been infected. They are all equipped with rubber gloves and goggles.

Education of inmates in the general prison population has been started by a nurse accompanied by an inmate who has AIDS. Bringing the message to eight thousand prisoners is no small chore. We attended one meeting open to all prisoners. Many prisoners were afraid of being identified as homosexual if they were to attend.

The state medical administration and some legislators are trying to require compulsory testing of all inmates. The Centers of Disease Control estimates that California men between the ages of twenty-nine and thirty would test positive at the rate of one in nine. If so, there are at least seven thousand seropositives in the California system. A higher-than-average incidence of drug needle users should boost this figure dramatically.

Judging by incidents at Vacaville and information from prisoners transferred from other prisons, education of both prisoners and staff elsewhere is nonexistent. There is talk of starting an organized effort. Education of prisoners will have little effect in slowing the spread of the disease within prisons unless it is accompanied by free issue of condoms and bleach (for needle cleaning), requiring a change in the law and regulations. This may happen when the public perceives the prisons as a main source of spreading the disease in the general population.

Living conditions for convicts assigned to the segregated AIDS areas have improved very slowly but steadily. Similar facilities will soon be activated in Southern California. This may place some inmates closer to their families. It may also relieve over-crowding in Vacaville temporarily. Yesterday there were only seven empty cots on a dual-occupancy basis. Improvements are due in part to an investiga-tion by the U.S. Department of Justice. Also some top administrators at Vacaville are genuinely interested and concerned.

We are interested in improving the plight of the convicts confined to the AIDS wings, the staff that deals with them, and the prison population as a whole. We participate in off-site stress-reduction ses-sions for the long-suffering staff. We are now treated by the old-time inmates as "part of the furniture," and with love and respect.

Cordially,
Nancy Jaicks and Bob Alexander

Epilogue

This is only the beginning.

The numbers show that the magnitude of AIDS in the United States, and the case load we can count on, is nothing less than staggering. By the end of 1991 an estimated 270,000 cases of AIDS will have occurred with 179,000 deaths within the decade since the disease was first recognized. In the year 1991 an estimated 145,000 patients with AIDS will need health and supportive services at a total cost of between $8 billion and $16 billion.

It is true that the work at San Francisco General Hospital serves as a model and will continue to do so—but what about the other hospitals in the cities and towns all across the country? I am reminded of the patient who tried to convince his doctor of the seriousness of his illness, only to be told not to worry, "It is just a rash." Or A., who was told by his physician, "You look great, you don't even need to get completely undressed. I'll listen to your heart—you know you're healthy." Then the patient took his shirt off and dropped his pants and he was covered with lesions. . . .

Or F., who came from New York to California and truly believed he was still alive only because he had been able to move out West:

> You know what the medical care in New York is like. I'd be dead by now if I'd stayed there. I've seen how even medical people refused to take care of AIDS patients. Just taking a verbal history from them, they refuse to do it. They brought me out here to San Francisco to the Shanti houses because AIDS people in New York had no support. . . . It's like night and day. They continually give the answer whenever you ask for anything, "Well look, we're overworked and understaffed."

Or the inmate who, prior to his incarceration, sought medical help for his growing concern about spreading Kaposi's sarcoma on his legs and was told, "Don't worry about it, they're just varicose veins." This is but one example, but I need hardly remind you of the overall state of our prisons, of the often insensitive, inhuman ways prisoners with AIDS are treated there.

Remember the same young patient whose K.S. had spread all over his body, and he begged the prison doctors to send him for some radiation or to a licensed hospital where treatment would be available to him. He was told he could only get the required necessary form once he was in the process of dying and he was not yet close to death. I wonder, had I not interceded on behalf of this man during my visit to the prison, if he would have ever been provided with any treatment at all for his ravaging disease.

Prisoners die in a sea of loneliness, locked up for months in isolation, deprived of books, TV, radio, or any physical exercise or fresh air. No wonder that, more than anything, they begged me to find them a pen pal so they could keep in touch with the outside world which appears to have abandoned them.

The most heartbreaking of all is the fate of the babies who are born with AIDS. It is like a recurring nightmare for me to think of these infants and toddlers dreadfully ill, neglected and rejected, with mothers too ill to take care of them. This is what is happening now to our innocent infants.

I have been so concerned about helping these children that I offered a piece of my farmland to create a small hospice here in Virginia for as many as I could handle. The outcry of the community was unimaginable. I was talked about and treated as if I were one of the witches of Salem. Only images of Jesus and Damien—both of whom worked with lepers—kept me going during those difficult years. So much hatred was stirred up by the thought of creating a safe and loving place for these tiny dying ones. While a few meager attempts to establish AIDS baby hospices are made in Northern California and Texas, too many of these children are doomed to spend their short life span in a hospital at great costs to taxpayers, being used as targets for research. They will never see the outdoors, a leaf or a flower, or take a stroll through a garden watching a butterfly. They need to be kissed, hugged, fondled and adored, with a permanent love object, not nurses around the clock (no matter how good a job they do).

For women and men with AIDS the story is sadly no different. They are rejected and stigmatized everywhere—by their fellow men, by their families, by their fellow workers, and even by their churches. What is even more disturbing is that the hospitals that are meant to treat them offer them, in most cases, minimal care. There are not enough doctors, there are not enough nurses, there are not enough support systems.

The gay community, which is the hardest hit with AIDS, has had to suffer by themselves in the lonely years when AIDS was first recognized and was considered a homosexual disease. They had to endure the worst kind of discrimination. Many of them have had to suffer in isolation. Some cannot tell their families. Some are even afraid to tell their doctors. Some cannot even face their friends. Who knows how many have committed suicide? How many AIDS sufferers have left their social setting and have gone, who knows where, to die alone. I, myself, have known of several single mothers and their infants who have done just that.

With such enormous prejudice against AIDS patients, and fear of them, people lose sight of the fact that most—if not almost all—die an early death at a time when their lives have just begun, when they are starting to make their contribution to society. The gay movement has tried to enlighten us about the enormous contributions of homosexuals to our society, but as far as AIDS is concerned, most of us are still in the Dark Ages.

If we are not careful the emergence of the AIDS epidemic will continue to polarize the population: a split between those who offer to help, and those who judge, label, and denigrate those afflicted. If we choose not to help persons with AIDS we will find ourselves with no hope for the future and no hope for mankind.

I pray that finally people will no longer see AIDS as a gay disease. I pray, too, that there will be a glimmer of hope in the emerging support systems that individuals like Irene and the Shanti groups and San Francisco General Hospital have organized in San Francisco.

But how many Irenes will we need? How many are prepared to play such a role and stick their necks out to help? How many are willing to be treated as if they had AIDS themselves? People like Irene have given dignity back to our patients. She has given them care, understanding, compassion, and love.

If we take our blinders off, we can see clearly the unimaginable task we have before us. The time has come to separate the wheat from the chaff: We have to choose between rejecting millions of our own because of their illness, or reaching out to offer help, warmth, and acceptance.

What are we to make of this hell of AIDS? Let us look again at the prophesies, from the Holy Scriptures, to the Hopi Indians, to Nostradamus. It has been foretold that there will be a time of great plague; there will be a time of the separation of the wheat from the chaff prior to great changes on this planet earth. We have also been taught, over endless time, that *love* is always stronger than anything else and can literally conquer all evil. If we are to believe all of this, wouldn't it be simple to spend our joint energies and resources (on every level) to organize a worldwide team, not only for research but for care centers, support groups, treatment centers, counseling centers, and bereavement groups?

It would create myriad jobs, a golden opportunity for lonesome old people, an educational chance for minorities, and a sense of working on a common goal toward a world family where men help for the betterment of mankind.

There would still be millions of dying young people on this planet Earth; AIDS will still decimate a large part of the population, but the quality of life would blossom, fear could be vanquished, love could flourish, service would be the purpose of life, and we would all learn to live up to a prayer that millions of us pray every night:

Our Father which art in heaven,
Hallowed be Thy name.
Thy kingdom come.
THY WILL BE DONE ON EARTH AS IT IS IN HEAVEN.
Give us this day our daily bread
And forgive us our debts, as we forgive our debtors.
And lead us not into temptation; but deliver us from evil:
For Thine is the kingdom, and the power, and the glory,
forever.
Amen.

Instead of viewing AIDS patients as being punished by God, is it not possible that they will eventually be viewed as the catalysts who set in motion these wonderful—and totally possible—world changes? I am reminded of the Second World War when my little country of Switzerland was totally surrounded by the bombing and destructiveness of the four world powers. We, the Swiss, have never felt such a sense of togetherness and solidarity as during the time of greatest national danger.

AIDS poses its own threat to mankind, but unlike war, it is a battle from within, knowing no borders or national boundaries. Are we going to choose hate and discrimination, or will we have the courage to choose love and service? Yes, I truly believe that AIDS is the ultimate challenge for all of us. Choose wisely, take the highest road you can, so that you will have no regrets at the end.

Blessings to all of you who are willing to serve and to love *unconditionally*.

—*Elisabeth*

Appendix

The Rising Cost of This Epidemic

The rising cost of this epidemic raises other, more important issues which our society and, for that matter, the rest of the world, has to face sooner or later. Medicine has not spent much energy and devotion in teaching people how to stay well and has developed few seminars and workshops in preventive medicine until very recently. The largest number of physicians either frown upon or openly ridicule patients who seek "other" kinds of treatment like visualization, acupuncture, acupressure, Bach remedies, etcetera, just to name a few.

We have learned from working with cancer patients how frustrated thousands of them are when they seek help (if not help, at least understanding, compassion, and partial relief), and when they seek treatments which do not fall into the orthodox medical model. Thousands have

had to save their hard-earned money to fly to places like
the Philippines or Mexico to receive alternative treatments, which helped some of their friends or neighbors.
We have been too long an arrogant bunch of scientists
who believed that we cannot do wrong and that we—and
only we—have all the answers. Naturally it has to be
stated that we earn our living by taking care of sick people
and unless there is some secondary gratification by keeping our patients well, maybe the majority of doctors will
never be enthusiastic spending their days with healthy
people (and only being reimbursed as long as they stay
healthy)!

AIDS has been a blow for many physicians, and it has
been a humiliating experience, first to have trouble diag-
nosing it, and then—after the early eighties—to acknowledge that there is very little they can do for their
patients. It was in the last one to two years that an increasing number of physicians have openly endorsed alternative treatments and many of them were grateful to
find a place for their patients that offered them increased comfort, if not improved health. A patient who
feels comfortable and not hopeless is much more cooper-
ative and grateful for the smallest service we can render
him/her!

In November 1985 health-care officials warned Congress that the costs of caring for AIDS patients threatened
to strain the Nation's hospitals, possibly forcing many of
them out of business. The first ten thousand patients spent
$6 billion in hospital bills, with a staggering amount of loss
of income. Since the greatest majority of these patients
are between the ages of twenty-five and forty-nine, with
extremely few cases in the retirement age, the loss of
potential work labor and work income is estimated at

$189 million. This would be computed at 8,370 years of work in potential lost earnings during their illnesses.

The Journal of the American Medical Association (January 86), states that for the first ten thousand patients, the average cost for hospital care was about $147,000. If the cases continue to double every nine to eleven months, it takes little knowledge in mathematics to realize that something has to be done soon before hospitals, hospices, and insurance institutions go bankrupt.

Studies from San Francisco, Philadelphia, and New York revealed that the average survival time between diagnosis and death is 392 days, of which, according to Dr. Ann Hardy from the Centers of Disease Control in Atlanta, estimates show that the average AIDS patient is hospitalized for 168 days prior to his death. Steven Gamble, president of the Hospital Council of Southern California, said that any hospital that cannot recover its costs from insurance, the government, or local taxpayers, either has to transfer the patients or close its doors. The public hospitals bear the biggest burden as they have always cared for the indigent patients. However, they will be unable to bear the responsibility of taking care of the increasing number of AIDS patients. Medicaid benefits often do not cover the total costs of the AIDS patients. An estimated 60 percent of the people with this disease are covered by Medicaid.

"Taxpayers in New York are expected to pay between $33 million and $45 million for AIDS patients at city-owned facilities," said Jo Ivey Boufford, acting president of the city's Health and Hospital Corporation.

The administrator of Glades General Hospital in Belle Glade, Florida, the "AIDS capitol of the United States," with more than one patient per one thousand population, pleaded for help for their seventy-three-bed hospital in order to remain financially solvent. So far, the Health Insurance Association of America has not demanded mandatory testing for new applicants of health insurance but made it clear that many firms would like to impose this restriction and would then deny coverage if a candidate would test HTLV-positive.

Health insurances are doubly at risk since the occurrence of tuberculosis will also add to their costs. With a weakened immune system, many of the AIDS patients are vulnerable to all sorts of infections, including TB. Dr. Dixie Snider, director of the Division of Tuberculosis Control at the Centers for Disease Control, stated that TB has decreased annually by 6 to 7 percent, and now has stopped decreasing with many AIDS patients also having tuberculosis. With over one million known carriers of the virus, she, as well as many others, is concerned that these HTLV-positive but otherwise symptom-free carriers can transmit it to family, friends, and health-care workers, if people are not tested for TB and treated before they contaminate others.

In *Lifelines,* the publication of the Life Foundation, we read of well-designed, free, anonymous, and voluntary testing for the HTLV-III antibodies for those persons who feel they will be helped to make behavioral changes to reduce the risk of transmission of the virus. This foundation believes that many people will be more motivated to follow the risk-reduction guidelines by knowing their antibody results, regardless of whether positive or negative. The foundation does not support mandatory testing of anyone, nor does it sanction testing which does not guarantee anonymity.

In March 1985, the Foundation, like many organizations on the mainland of the United States, took a strong stand against the use of the HTLV-III Ab test for any purpose other than what the test was originally designed for; namely, screening of blood and blood products at blood banks. At that time: 1) there was inadequate understanding of the test's use in the clinical/diagnostic environment; 2) there was fear of false results; and 3) there was a significant potential for the creation and abuse of lists of high risk individuals who chose to take the test. Adequate legal safeguards were not in place, and are still not guaranteed in this country, in contrast to Switzerland, for example, where the total and absolute confidentiality is guaranteed between physician and patient!

In the subsequent year, many things have happened, of which the public is not always aware. The Foundation has since offered free testing in an anonymous environment and points out that individuals who had the tests taken in a private doctor's office have had their insurance canceled in spite of the fact that they were perfectly healthy and showed a negative test!

With a worldwide, extremely costly epidemic like this one, we have to review and reevaluate many areas of our daily existence. We can no longer continue the health-care system, to which we were accustomed. We can no longer take it for granted that we will have a hospital bed available when we need one. We can no longer be sure that a health insurance is available to us which covers the cost, if we should have a lengthy and, perhaps, terminal illness. We can no longer have our egos and profits in the way of human services. We can no longer lay claim to being the only people who can take good care of patients as long as we have an M.D. degree. And last, but equally important, maybe we will learn to live more in the *now* instead of spending 90 percent of our energies in worrying about tomorrow. We may need to look at our own lives, our own values, and learn to share more of our own resources in order to assure that everybody has enough in times of health, and in times of illness.

One of the best models of care for AIDS patients comes from San Francisco, where a whole ward has been dedicated to AIDS patients exclusively, and where an increasing number of trained Shanti volunteers have taken over a great many hours of home care and necessary adjunct treatments of these patients. Much more effort has to be put into resources for all AIDS patients, from little rejected babies of IV drug-using mothers to a great number of unemployable young men who are too sick to earn a living and not so sick and in imminent need of medical facilities, to house them, feed them, nurture them physically, emotionally, and spiritually. They are too young to have saved up enough money for the time of their retirement; many have been dropped from their insurances and too many have been rejected by their own families and friends who would ordinarily take care of them if it were for any other disease but AIDS!

Ostracized and often rejected and alone, indigent and sick, many of them have resorted to suicide a couple of years ago. In San Francisco, where there is a model support system, this is far less of a problem than anywhere else in the U.S. Twenty-four-hour answering services are available and thousands of hours of counseling, massage therapy and support have been given to these patients without charge, when they could not afford it.

As early as 1985, I visited the Centers for Disease Control and offered not only to set up programs to train "an army of volunteers" nationwide to take over these tasks, but I also offered the opening of Hospices for Children with AIDS.* With between six hundred to three thousand** children with AIDS in the country, many without families or caring next of kin, they are kept in hospitals at enormous costs, and are easy targets for research and financial gain, instead of being housed with loving caring families and the pleasure of playmates, pets, fresh air, and a garden for the short time they still have to enjoy being on this planet.

When money, politics, and ego get into the way of the care of our patients, the whole country should stand up and say, "NO"! We call ourselves a "mainly Christian country," but we surely don't practice it consistantly!

It should be viewed as a privilege to help our fellow man, to serve as we would like to be served if we should ever get sick and/or indigent, and we should regard it a privilege to take into our homes these pitiful children, truly victims of a society which has lost much of its early pioneering spirit and willingness to love unconditionally and serve without expectation of reward.

---

*See "Children and AIDS."
**Many live "underground" and have never been reported.

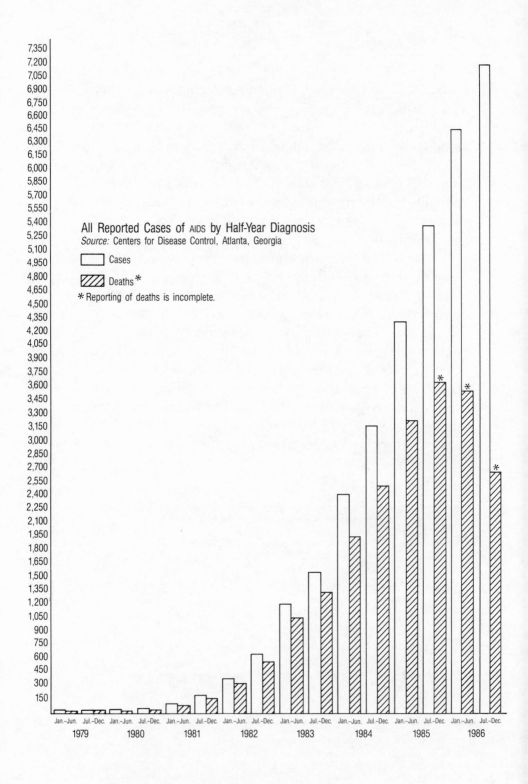

All Reported Cases of AIDS by Half-Year Diagnosis
Source: Centers for Disease Control, Atlanta, Georgia

☐ Cases

▨ Deaths*

* Reporting of deaths is incomplete.